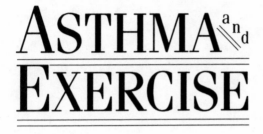

ASTHMA and EXERCISE

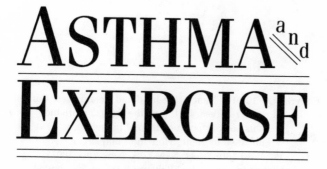

ASTHMA and
EXERCISE

Nancy Hogshead and
Gerald Secor Couzens

HENRY HOLT AND COMPANY
New York

Published by Henry Holt and Company, Inc.,
115 West 18th Street, New York, New York 10011.
Published in Canada by Fitzhenry & Whiteside Limited,
195 Allstate Parkway, Markham, Ontario L3R 4T8.

LIBRARY OF CONGRESS CATALOGING-IN-PUBLICATION DATA
Hogshead, Nancy.
Asthma and exercise / Nancy Hogshead and Gerald Secor Couzens.—
1st ed.
p.   cm.
Includes index.
ISBN 0-8050-0878-0
1. Asthma.   2. Exercise.   3. Asthmatics—Rehabilitation.
I. Couzens, Gerald Secor.   II. Title.
RC591.H63   1989
616.2'38—dc20   89-7615
                                                              CIP

Henry Holt books are available at special discounts
for bulk purchases for sales promotions, premiums,
fund-raising, or educational use. Special editions
or book excerpts can also be created to specification.

For details contact:

Special Sales Director
Henry Holt and Company, Inc.
115 West 18th Street
New York, New York 10011

First Edition

Designed by Kathryn Parise
Printed in the United States of America
1   3   5   7   9   10   8   6   4   2

CONTENTS

ACKNOWLEDGMENTS

This book is, above all, a resource book, and it couldn't have been written without the help of the many athletes we interviewed. We are indebted to all of these fine people, who gave of their time not only to relay their own asthma stories, but also to offer personal tips that will help in the exercise routines and training of others. These athletes are: Jill Abrams, Jim Angel, Keith Brantley, Joe Carabino, Christine Dakin, Bruce Davidson, Shirley Dery-Batlik, Anita DeFrantz, Rick DeMont, Cheryl Durstein-Decker, Virginia Gilder, Mike Gminski, Alexi Grewal, Jackie Joyner-Kersee, Bill Koch, Greg Louganis, Danny Manning, George Murray, Rob Muzzio, Joe Nieder, Doug Padilla, Joan Pennington, Sam Perkins, Pat Porter, John Powell, Jim Ryun, Sandra Samberg, Manuel Sanguily, Michael Secrest, Karin K. Smith, Tracy Sundlund, Bonnie Warner, and James Wofford.

We are indebted, too, to William E. Pierson, M.D., nationally known authority on asthma and exercise, who reviewed the book and made suggestions. Leo Leonidas, M.D., editor of the *Asthma Today* newsletter, was also extremely helpful in reviewing the book and offering advice and medical comments.

We would also like to thank the following physicians and scientists for their thoughts and advice: Robert Fuentes, doctor of pharmacy, who provided invaluable asthma research; Francois

Haas, Ph.D., who has studied exercise and asthma in his New York lab; Steven Jonas, M.D., an "ordinary mortal" athlete who contributed to the walking section; Roger Katz, M.D., clinical professor of pediatrics, UCLA School of Medicine, who treats many top athletes who have asthma; Henry Milgrom, M.D., who works with children regularly at the National Jewish Center for Immunology and Respiratory Medicine in Denver; David M. Orenstein, M.D., of Children's Hospital of Pittsburgh, who directed the child asthma exercise study; and James Rippe, M.D., director of the exercise physiology lab at the University of Massachusetts Medical Center, who contributed to the walking section.

We are grateful also to Lori Boniface, for the story of her son, Danny; to Bob Anderson for his stretching pointers; and to Ian Jackson for his BreathPlay techniques. To Louann Exum and Tom Williams, we owe our deepest gratitude for sharing their personal stories of sorrow so that countless others might benefit.

We are especially indebted to Channa Taub of Henry Holt and Company for her patience and understanding, especially on that hot summer afternoon when she helped steer the book in another direction. Thanks, Channa, for your skillful and intelligent editing. Thanks, of course, to literary agent Jim Trupin, who put us together with Channa. And a special thanks to Frank Michel, who tirelessly tracked down many of our interviewees and helped give shape and body to the text from start to finish. The photographs of Nancy exercising and the illustrations were done by Elisa and Rosemary Michel, and John Bonis of Articles, Inc., in New York. We thank them for their excellent work.

Nancy Hogshead
Gerald Secor Couzens
New York City
April 1989

Writing this book was all too often a lonely affair, and through it all my wife, Elisa, was understanding and always there with endless encouragement, especially during those crunch times that meant yet another late night. Thanks, Elisa.

G.S.C.

Without my swimming coaches, Randy Reese, Bob Thompson, and Mitch Ivey, my swimming talent would have never been recognized, encouraged, or have flourished, and I thank them for the lessons they taught me—ones I am still using.

Gil Mott of Allen & Hamburys Division of Glaxo, Inc., has wholeheartedly supported my education and involvement with asthmatics these past five years. Without his belief in me, his allowance for my mistakes, my involvement with asthmatics couldn't be what it is today.

Nancy Sander, founder and president of Mothers of Asthmatics, Inc., is one of my first resources for practical information on living with asthma and how to communicate effectively with health care professionals, asthmatics and their families, and the public.

Last, I would like to thank my parents, Janet and Howard Hogshead, for their unerring support and encouragement for my life's passions.

N.H.

FOREWORD

Asthma and Exercise is a long-overdue book. Gone are the days when a person with asthma had to stay on the sidelines, held back from participation in exercise or sports, whether on the recreational, competitive, or world-class level. Now we know that exercise benefits everyone—and that with proper guidance those with asthma may participate in and fully enjoy exercise and sports activities.

Asthma, caused by hyperresponsive airways, affects about 10 million children and adults, but many don't recognize the symptoms. Many athletes, coaches, parents, and even doctors will often attribute the symptoms of asthma, such as difficulty in breathing or a constant cough, to the person's being out of shape or having yet another cold. This book helps people to recognize asthma, seek treatment, and gain control of their health. It also explores all the benefits of exercise for people with asthma: Exercise helps build cardiopulmonary fitness, boosts self-esteem, and improves overall health. The end result is often better management of the condition.

This book contains the latest asthma medical advances and has many resources for people with asthma to draw upon. Its most outstanding feature, however, is the personal stories of the athletes who have achieved athletic success in spite of their asthma. Many of these athletes have had asthma for years, but with effective medical attention they were able to rise to the highest athletic standards. Their inspiring stories and practical tips should be of great benefit in motivating people with asthma not only to seek proper medical treatment, but also to exercise and compete in sports.

We congratulate the authors for this important and practical book. We believe that it will help provide you or your child with the vital information needed to successfully treat and manage asthma and will help you reap the benefits that exercise and sports offer.

William E. Pierson, M.D.
Clinical Professor, Pediatrics and Environmental Health,
University of Washington, Seattle

Robert O. Voy, M.D.
Former Chief Medical Officer and Director of Sports
  Medicine and Science,
United States Olympic Committee

A SPECIAL NOTE

When you think of asthma, what comes to mind? How would you describe asthma? Many people would use the following phrases to describe the condition: "I suffer from asthma"; "Asthma attacks my lungs"; "I'm an asthma cripple"; "I'm having an asthma attack."

Now, try substituting these phrases for the ones above: "I have asthma"; "Asthma affects my lungs"; "I'm having some asthma"; "I'm having an asthma episode."

The first group of phrases is the language of a victim, and you will notice that those terms are not used in this book. Those phrases conjure up an image of an anxious person who is helplessly waiting for his next case of asthma to swoop down and incapacitate him.

At one time there was very little that people with asthma could do to help themselves, and they probably had a credible claim to calling themselves victims. But today, after all the many medical breakthroughs in asthma research, no one has to remain a victim any longer. With peak-flow meters and an understanding of allergens and other asthma triggers, asthma can be predicted. By taking medicines and using breathing exercises, asthma can be controlled.

Unfortunately, the language we use to describe asthma has been much slower to change than the treatment of asthma. The way we talk about asthma usually defines how we experience it, including how much or how little control we feel we have over our fate.

Asthma researchers have found that if people with asthma feel they have no control over their condition, they often will not respond to the earliest asthma signals until it's too late and they are seriously ill. Therefore, the first step in changing how we feel about asthma is to change the way we talk about it.

Language is a powerful tool, and therefore we must be especially mindful of how asthma is discussed in front of children with asthma. Impressions of the self formed early in life are often permanent, so by taking a positive approach to asthma, stressing that asthma is controllable and manageable and that in most cases children with asthma can participate in all sports, we'll be doing the best we can to ensure that those children will grow up feeling competent, with a healthy self-image, and able to accomplish whatever their goals might be.

TO OUR READERS

From time to time in the book we recommend that you consult your physician in a variety of situations. This book is designed to guide and educate those who have asthma. Often in the life of a person with asthma a doctor is helpful and necessary. It is wise to consult with a doctor before undertaking an exercise program, changing your diet, taking any kind of medication, or selecting a place to live. So, while we hope this book will help you, it should not be used as a substitute for sound medical advice.

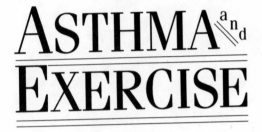

ASTHMA and EXERCISE

1

ASTHMA: HOW IT AFFECTED MY LIFE

Breathing: in with the good air, out with the bad. For most, it's that simple. However, for the millions of Americans who have asthma (many of whom are unaware of their condition), breathing can often become conscious and labored. This doesn't have to be the case, though. In fact, there are few limits to what people with asthma can achieve once they are properly diagnosed, begin medication, and start to get their asthma under control. That's what I've learned from my own experience, although for years I never even knew I had asthma.

From 1974 to 1984, when I was a competitive swimmer, I would sometimes feel unusually winded and tired during my workouts and competitions. After some particularly hard training session or race, it wasn't uncommon for me to pass out momentarily at poolside or have my face turn purple from exertion. I regarded this as normal, something brought on by going all out. After all, pushing yourself to the limit will often leave you breathless.

I'd think I was simply working harder than my teammates and competitors. My coaches thought it was terrific when I passed out, and they praised my "toughness." All the while I associated my heavy breathing with "not being in shape" or told myself that this was evidence that I was pushing the envelope of my physical limitations. I attributed most of my difficulties to physical or mental training defects and scolded myself for not working hard enough in practice or for not being tough enough at the end of a race.

I generally came down with a whooping case of bronchitis once a year, but it never occurred to me that my breathing difficulties were linked to asthma. None of the coaches I trained with or physicians who examined me during that period ever indicated I had a special breathing problem. The word *asthma* was certainly never mentioned. Then, in 1984, things changed abruptly and I discovered that my breathing problems were not all in my head.

Participating in the Olympic Games is the thrill of a lifetime, and my family and I were really looking forward to the 200-meter butterfly final at the Los Angeles Games in 1984. With my three golds and one silver, I had already won more medals than any other swimmer in the Games. With a medal in this, my last race, I could tie the record for the most medals won in women's Olympic swimming competition.

The 200-meter butterfly, four laps in the 50-meter pool, is a grueling race because the mechanics of the stroke demand so much strength, coordination, endurance, and oxygen. While I can swim miles freestyle in practice without any difficulty, just one continuous butterfly mile is enough to exhaust me.

From the moment the starter's gun sounded, all went perfectly. However, with only 20 meters to go, my breathing suddenly became labored, and, without enough oxygen, my arms felt heavy. Swimmers jokingly call this feeling "the bear that jumped on my back."

Here I was in the best shape of my life, yet I found myself gasping for air in order to reach the end of the pool. I floundered and the other swimmers outtouched me at the wall. I finished in fourth place, disappointed, and just .07 second away from the bronze medal.

I got out of the pool coughing and wheezing and then went to a special area to gather my belongings. I happened to meet a volunteer Olympic physician there who asked if I always coughed so heavily after swimming. I proudly responded yes, since I thought the cough was proof positive that I had really gone for it in the race.

The doctor invited me to a nearby lab for a treadmill test. I was

immediately interested, not least of all because I had done exceptionally well on every other test I had taken leading up to the
Olympics. This would be another opportunity for me to demonstrate how all my years of intensive swim training had helped make
me an outstanding athlete. Or so I thought.

Several days later I took the test, which consisted of running on
a treadmill at gradually increasing speeds. When it was over the
doctor announced, "You have exercise-induced bronchospasm.
Didn't you ever notice that you have trouble breathing when you
exert yourself in exercise?"

I was stunned and thought that the man was crazy. "That's just
not possible," I told him quite adamantly. "There must be a mistake. Me? Asthma? Didn't you see me swim?"

I listened as the doctor ticked off a number of asthma symptoms,
and I started replaying in my mind many of the difficult breathing
incidents I had had during my career, incidents I had ascribed to
being "out of shape" (this from someone who swam up to eight
hundred laps a day!) or not trying hard enough or being born with
small lungs.

Those weren't the reasons at all, I was now being told. In a way,
I felt relieved because I finally had a name and a medical diagnosis
for something I had been living with for a long time.

I remembered that my breathing problems had first surfaced
when I was fourteen. I had put on a lot of muscle because of my
increased training load and weight lifting, and I thought my breathing problems were due to nothing more than the added muscle.
Even though my older brother Andy—an outstanding athlete who
rowed on the varsity crew team at Harvard—had asthma and took
daily medication, it never entered my mind that my breathing
difficulty was similar to his. Besides, he was allergic to just about
everything imaginable and I had no allergies.

The first time I passed out in practice was when I was sixteen
years old and I can recall saying to myself, "I've got to learn how
to breathe faster. I have to concentrate more." My wheezing and
coughing didn't go unnoticed by my coaches. When I got older,
one of them took me aside and started working with me on an
exercise that consisted of taking a series of deep, controlled breaths,

a form of hyperventilation. "You're a big girl and you're going to need the extra oxygen at the end of the race," he said. He was aware of my need for "extra oxygen," but like me, he had no idea what this need stemmed from.

Swimming as a sport has its own unique challenges. In addition to logging as many as thirteen miles a day, putting in hours of weight lifting, and doing hundreds of sit-ups and push-ups, swimmers work specifically on exercising without breathing. This is called "hypoxic training" and is meant to build up lung capacity and endurance. A swimmer wants to be as streamlined as possible as he or she strokes through the water, and while you do need to breathe, every time you move your head to breathe in air, you change body position, creating drag and slowing down a bit. By cutting down on the number of breaths you take during a race, you can very often improve your overall time.

The farthest I ever swam without breathing was one and three-quarters Olympic pool lengths, or just over three lengths of a high-school pool. This happened right after completing a set of several 50-meter hypoxic sprints. I had been working out that day with Billy Forrester, 1976 bronze medalist in the 200-meter butterfly, and John Hillencamp, national silver medalist in the 1,500 meters. After our regular workout, both fellows announced that they were going to try to swim an additional 100 meters without breathing. Even though my head still hurt from the hypoxic drills, I could sense the challenge and intensity in their voices and my competitive juices began flowing. I made up my mind to match them stroke for stroke.

It hurts to swim without breathing, and after 50 meters my lungs were burning. But I could see that Billy and John had stopped at about the 65-meter mark and I wanted to go farther. I made it all the way to 80 meters, but by then my head was spinning and I suddenly blacked out in the pool. Later, after being carried to the pool deck where I woke up, I started giggling because I knew that I had gone the farthest. This may not have been the most mature thing I've ever done in my life, but I've always found it hard to resist a challenge.

Despite a steady diet of these rigorous practice sessions, I still felt exceptionally winded at the end of a race and my rib cage often felt as sore as my biceps. At such times I would resolve to work harder and try to become as emotionally tough and competitive as possible in order to compensate for what I now thought were my "small lungs." If only they were "bigger," I told myself, I would be able to breathe in more air.

I was convinced that nature had shortchanged me in the lung department, and that if I wanted to be a top swimmer, I had no choice but to work on it. My "small lung" theory allowed me to ignore the fact that something was seriously wrong.

Prior to the 1984 Olympics, all the American athletes were administered a battery of physical and mental tests by our team physicians. These ranged from gauging the strength of our pull to electronically plotting our strokes on a computer to test for efficiency. I still remember the medical test for my blood lactate level, which measured the amount of waste product in my bloodstream. The results came back very high. This was not uncommon for someone who had just finished a difficult, intense race, but I hadn't. My short practice swims were aimed at keeping me at only 70 percent of maximum effort.

The test results should have alerted someone that I wasn't getting enough oxygen and that my system was producing too much waste product and going into an anaerobic (exercising without oxygen) state too soon. This was hardly normal for an athlete as highly trained as myself, but it somehow failed to raise any red flags for me or for the doctors.

I continued to have difficulties with my breathing, but by rationalizing that I had smaller lungs than any of my teammates, and by failing to recognize the symptoms of asthma, I effectively kept myself from seeking medical help. When I was eventually given a standard pulmonary function test at the Olympic Training Center in 1984, I found out for the first time that my lung muscles were unusually strong and that I actually had a large lung capacity. As a matter of fact, my scores on the test that measured how much air I could move in and out of my lungs in thirty seconds were one-third higher than those of all the other Olympic female swimmers.

I was surprised by this finding, but I still failed to put two and two together. Forced now to abandon my theory about small lungs, I soon came up with another idea to explain away my fatigue, coughing, and passing out. I simply told myself that perhaps my cardiovascular system—which transfers oxygen through the bloodstream to the working muscles—was inefficient. Since I possessed strength, endurance, flexibility, and efficient strokes, it had to be my cardiovascular system that was the weak link.

As fate would have it, every test I was given before the Olympics was while I was at rest. If I had been exercising vigorously for as little as six to eight minutes prior to the test, my exercise-induced bronchospasm (EIB) would have been detected and I would have been given medicine and learned all the necessary procedures to control asthma.

Shortly after my post-Olympic treadmill test, I was given albuterol to try. Albuterol is a beta-adrenergic bronchodilator that helps relax the muscle surrounding the air passages and open clogged bronchial tubes. When used before exercise it can prevent an asthma flare-up. I started with the medication in pill form but quickly switched to an inhaler. The inhaled medication contains only one-twentieth the medication of one pill, but that was all I needed to bring my condition under control before exercising.

I was astounded by how I felt during and after a workout. Taking just two puffs before a workout made an incredible difference. Exercising without medication now reminded me of swimming with two swimsuits on (something we often did in practice sessions to make us stronger swimmers; the extra suit makes it difficult to swim fast by increasing water resistance). Exercising after taking the medication made me feel as if I had "shaved down" (shaving the body outside the swimsuit reduces drag and increases sensitivity to the water) and was wearing a racing suit. With the medication I was amazed that people could breathe this easily, so effortlessly, all the time, even when they were really pouring it on in a workout!

I know that you can't go back and change history, but if I had only known about my asthma sooner, things just might have been different in that last Olympic race in 1984. Not only would I have been able to get more oxygen while competing, but I would have been able to work out on a daily basis at a much higher level.

Controlling my asthma now is a relatively simple matter. Twenty minutes before I go to exercise, I take my two puffs from an albuterol inhaler (Ventolin), put my hair in a braid, lace up my sneakers, and then I'm out the door to dance classes, off for a run or a bike ride in the park, or over to the pool for some lap swimming. I also enjoy tennis, water skiing, wind surfing, and snow skiing, all without the bother of asthma because I now know my symptoms and how to keep them under control.

My asthma hasn't diminished in any way over the years and actually seems to get worse whenever I begin to lose my physical conditioning. I know that I'll probably be taking medication before exercising for the rest of my life, but I'm realistic enough to know that should I ever forget to take my medication, I could be bent over with severe coughing and left with a pair of very sore lungs that will bother me for some time afterward. Thinking about that is reminder enough to take my medication.

ASTHMA SPOKESPERSON

After the Olympics my life took some twists and turns that I certainly never expected. I had always planned to finish my undergraduate degree and go on to law school. That's not exactly what happened.

During the four hectic weeks following the Games I was asked to speak before different groups on a variety of topics. I began giving motivational speeches to large companies, relating excellence in the sports arena to achievement in the business world. With the help of the Women's Sports Foundation, I spoke to journalists, and went on radio and television to speak about Title IX, the landmark legislation requiring more sports and athletic opportunities be made available for females. Title IX was directly responsible for my athletic scholarship at Duke University, and certainly for my continued interest in sports at the age of twenty-two. Without Title IX, I would surely have had to curtail my sports participation after high school, because there simply wouldn't have been any collegiate sports activities geared for women. Without those activities, there would be mostly fifteen- and sixteen-year-olds at the Olympics representing the United States and not as many twenty- to twenty-four-year-olds as you see now.

I also addressed the Republican National Convention on the pride that all Americans can feel when our athletes compete in the Olympics. On another occasion I spoke before Congress about the importance of sports and fitness for our youth, not only for the obvious health benefits, but also for the socialization skills and opportunities that sports can offer.

I have always believed that participation in sports has numerous social benefits, that the lessons boys and girls learn through sports will help them throughout their lives. At a very young age I learned how to be part of a team, how to set goals and achieve them, how to postpone short-term gratification for long-term rewards, how to win, and, just as important, how to lose with grace. You certainly don't have to be the best athlete in the world to learn these things and to have fun while doing so.

Sports has so much to offer everyone, including those with asthma. For Bonnie Warner, a 1984 and 1988 winter Olympian, grade school and high school in Upland, California, were times of trial because of asthma, but she found participating in sports a way of challenging herself and a great way to build confidence and self-esteem. "To a great extent, I am who I am because of sports. In addition, sports has helped my asthma," says Warner, a luge specialist whose asthma now is occasionally triggered by cats, smog, and cold weather, especially at high altitude.

Like an unexpected fast break, Danny Manning's first major bout with asthma came one day in the university gym, but just as the talented basketball star learned to handle all of the opponents who would double- and triple-team him throughout his successful collegiate career at the University of Kansas, he also learned how to manage his asthma. "Sports has put me through college, let me travel the world, and allowed me to meet a lot of interesting people," said Manning, the 6 foot 10, 1987–1988 NCAA College Basketball Player of the Year. "I never once thought my asthma would keep me from achieving anything. Once I started using the medication, I was certain that I would start to play even better." Shortly after Manning led the University of Kansas Jayhawks to the 1988 National Championship, he was selected number one in the NBA college draft by the Los Angeles Clippers.

The beauty of sports is that you learn by participating, competing, and sharing with others. "You also learn all about your own limitations," says Anita DeFrantz, who had asthma during childhood and went on to become a 1976 bronze medal–winning oarswoman at the Montreal Olympics and, soon after, a member of the International Olympic Committee. "Sports also lets you keep pushing at the borders of your limitations, in many cases pushing them back further. In doing so, children especially can develop greater lung capacity, and in many cases, not be so set back by asthma."

Although my competitive swim career is now over, I know that my sports and athletic experiences have made me much better equipped for whatever I choose to tackle in life. I'm sure the lessons I learned from years of training and competing can be applied to almost anything that lies ahead.

In the past few years I've spoken on the importance of sports and exercise not only to general audiences, but also to scores of asthma groups, made up of doctors, nurses, teachers, school administrators, entire middle schools and high schools, physical therapists, respiratory therapists, professional and amateur athletes, adult asthmatics, asthmatic children, and families of asthmatics. I've also spoken at dozens of asthma fund-raisers, medical meetings, and to television, radio, and newspapers about asthma and exercise.

Of all the groups, I receive the most pleasure in speaking to people who have asthma themselves. Most are interested not only in getting their condition under control, but in finding ways of participating in all life has to offer. Most want down-to-earth practical advice, solutions, and tips about how to handle their asthma. Many are highly motivated to try new approaches.

One thing, however, always bothered me in speaking about asthma. I've found that people with asthma, including kids, are the most sedentary group I've ever encountered. Because of their inactive ways (some self-imposed, others on doctors' or parents' orders), many were being left out of all the benefits—and the fun— of sports. How could I help remedy this?

I started by generally recommending that all people with asthma exercise, whether it be walking, swimming, running, bicycling, hiking, playing raquetball, football, or taking part in dance. Initially, many people in the audience were surprised because they had always heard advice to the contrary. "Doesn't exercise produce asthma?" was a typical question. Many kids used their asthma as a perfect way to avoid phys ed class at school. Parents would tell me that they'd feel better if they could let their children "outgrow" their asthma before starting them on any kind of athletic program. Some people with asthma simply shrugged their shoulders in resignation. "How can I ever participate in sports?" they'd say, and quickly rattle off a long list of medications they were taking.

The medical community's fairly recent about-face regarding exercise—it is now agreed that people with asthma should exercise if at all possible—has taken some time to trickle down to the general public. Too much time. That is where the inspiration for this book began.

I want to teach people with asthma how to exercise safely so that they can learn to control their asthma and put it on the back burner of their lives instead of keeping it the focal point. With their asthma properly managed, they can be free to fulfill their hopes and ambitions in whatever fields they choose.

When I speak about asthma, most people are surprised to learn of the new possibilities open to them. The excitement builds during my talk as I pass around one of my Olympic gold medals for them to look at. For some people with asthma, it's the first time they've allowed themselves to believe that they don't have to let asthma run their lives and that, despite asthma, the potential for an Olympic gold medal (or whatever their dream might be) is within reach.

ASTHMA AND EXERCISE

Get excited! The inspiring stories of the many Olympic and world-class athletes with asthma will show you that exercise is a powerful medication in its own right, one that can help people gain a sense of mastery over their bodies, a sense of control over their asthma and their lives. From sandbox to sandlot, from the jogging trail in the local park to the oval track at the Olympic stadium, these athletes with asthma have all been diagnosed and are currently under treatment. Yet they're able to play, exercise, work out, and compete with nonasthmatic athletes in spite of what some call a "disability." If you follow their workouts and suggestions, your life can also be enhanced.

You, too, can find an activity that will be both appropriate and enjoyable for you. The goal, after all, is *participation* in fitness activities, not necessarily an Olympic gold medal. But who knows . . . that just might be waiting for you also.

EXERCISE AND ASTHMA

Exercise can be for everyone, although not everyone gets excited by the idea. Why should you exercise, especially if you have asthma? Simply because health and fitness can be greatly improved by regular exercise, just as they can be for people without asthma. Not only will well-planned weekly workouts improve your cardiopulmonary (heart and lungs) health, aid in increasing bone density (actually making bones thicken and get stronger), reduce serum cholesterol (the levels of fat in your blood), and lower both your blood sugar and blood pressure levels, but in many cases they will also increase your feeling of well-being and raise your self-confidence.

The question many people ask first about asthma and exercise is whether a regular exercise program can actually reduce asthma symptoms or lessen the severity of a flare-up. Asthma researchers have been grappling with this question for years and it remains a controversial issue. Some research and anecdotal evidence indicates that exercise can reduce asthma symptoms, but other research says that it can't. From my own experience, I know that I need to exercise regularly to ward off asthma.

David M. Orenstein, M.D., a pediatric pulmonologist who treats

12

children with lung problems at Children's Hospital of Pittsburgh, is a great believer in the value of exercise for people with asthma and regularly helps develop exercise routines for his patients. However, Orenstein, who in 1985 conducted one of the first scientific studies to see if children with asthma who undertook a reasonable exercise conditioning program could become more fit and do so safely, does not believe that exercise will "cure" or lessen asthma severity.

In Orenstein's study, "Exercise Conditioning in Children with Asthma," twenty-three children with asthma, six to sixteen years of age, who required long-term oral or aerosolized bronchodilator therapy were divided into a control and an exercise group. Before the program got under way, both groups were tested on a bicycle ergometer to find their heart and lung capacities.

After this testing, the control group continued with their normal activities for the next four months, while the exercise group began a conditioning program that lasted one hour, three times a week. Each session had four phases: warm-up, endurance, cool-down, and fun.

The warm-up consisted of passing a basketball around with the hands or feet for five to ten minutes. The endurance phase, which consisted of walking-jogging-walking, was ten minutes long for the first week's sessions and then lengthened by two minutes per session each week thereafter, so that in the final, tenth-week sessions, the group was exercising for thirty uninterrupted minutes at 75 percent of maximal effort.

While the final results of the Orenstein research did not show a change in asthma severity in either the exercise or the control group, it did show that the exercise group had significant improvement in all responses to exercise: They had increased physical working capacity, higher peak oxygen consumption levels, and a decreased heart rate when they had to perform simple physical tasks.

Does this mean their asthma was "improved?" "The only way we define asthma improvement scientifically is with a peak-flow meter [a device for measuring peak expiratory flow rate]," says Dr. Orenstein. "And in our testing of the exercise group and the nonexercise group, the daily peak-flow measurements didn't change significantly in either group." However, notes Orenstein, the exercisers had more efficient breathing and could handle asthma symptoms much better.

Orenstein's clinical findings don't mean that people with asthma shouldn't exercise or that people with asthma don't benefit from exercise. "While I'm a believer in the notion that exercise programs do not help improve asthma per se, I feel very strongly that our data point out that exercise programs don't hurt a person with asthma and that exercise is so beneficial in so many other areas that it should not be avoided."

While doctors say that exercise won't cure asthma, there are many athletes like myself who report that their asthma seems more of a problem whenever they're in less than optimum physical condition. Dr. Orenstein explains that this happens because of one's breathing abilities. "The more fit you are and the more you exercise," says Orenstein, "the less strenuously you have to breathe for certain physical tasks because your cardiorespiratory system is now more efficient. You don't need as much air nor do you gasp for breath."

Dr. Orenstein doesn't recommend exercise to "cure" a person's asthma. "If you look to exercise for this reason, then forget it," he says. "But there are lots of other benefits that exercise gives you." Orenstein maintains that a regular exercise program will help a person with asthma to become more fit, to be able to accomplish goals, and to feel good about himself.

"I tell my patients that exercise certainly won't cure them of their asthma, but that it's not going to make their asthma any worse. It's also going to enable them to add another part to their life that had been closed off because of their reluctance to exercise. By becoming fit you can derive the same enjoyment that other kids and adults without asthma are able to get from exercise.

"If you look at the inherent properties of the bronchi and the muscles around the bronchi [see chapter 3] and how 'twitchy' they are and likely to go into spasm, it's my belief that this isn't changed by exercise," says Orenstein. According to Orenstein, the stimulus, the insult that you present to the bronchi in the form of cold or dry air, may actually be greater if you are less fit. Take in large volumes of air, says Orenstein, especially cold or dry air, and it is more likely that this will cause the air passages to go into spasm. However, if you are more fit, then you don't have to breathe quite so hard and the effect on the lungs will be reduced.

The work of Dr. Orenstein and his colleagues has clearly demonstrated that young patients with asthma who are given appropriate bronchodilators before exercising can safely and successfully complete a running program with the same increased fitness and work tolerance expected from nonasthmatics. Says Dr. Orenstein: "We urge physicians caring for young asthmatic patients to encourage them to take advantage of exercise opportunities and not to let the fear of exercise-induced asthma prevent them from leading a full, active life."

What can exercise do for a person with asthma? The way Dr. Manuel Sanguily sees things, he never had much choice in the matter. "Because of my asthma, I was a puny, rotten kid," he says. "Everyone thought I was going to die. I started swimming as a way to improve my prospects for survival."

Sanguily not only has kept up with his swimming, but has filled the record books with his accomplishments. Today, at age fifty-five, the Cuba-born Sanguily is a physician in family practice and sports medicine in Tarrytown, New York. Six days a week he logs 4,500 yards in the pool (just under three miles), working out at lunchtime and before and after office hours. That training, combined with some weight lifting, keeps him in top shape for the full schedule of Masters swim meets (for swimmers over the age of twenty-five) he competes in every year.

Since joining the Masters Association Swim Program in 1978 after a self-imposed twenty-year layoff from competitive swimming, Dr. Sanguily has won an impressive fifty national championships and set seven Masters world records in three different age groups. In eleven years of competition, he has yet to lose a single event in his specialty, the breaststroke. And every Labor Day, Sanguily swims the four miles across the Hudson River in New York "just for the fun of it."

As a young man, Sanguily represented Cuba in the 1952 and

1956 Olympic Games as well as the 1954 Central American Games, where he won a gold medal, and the 1955 Pan American Games, where he won a silver. In 1955, he entered medical school at Ohio State but still found time to train and compete.

"I'm a bulldog achiever," admits Sanguily. "I won't let my asthma keep me back." Between 1956 and 1959 he won a total of seven National U.S.A. Championships and in 1958 he set a world record in the 100-meter breaststroke with a time of 1:13:04.

Despite his numerous athletic accomplishments and severe asthma, Sanguily is always on the prowl for new challenges. In 1987 he decided to swim down the Hudson River from the Tappan Zee Bridge in Westchester County to the George Washington Bridge in Manhattan, some fifteen miles, in an effort to raise money and generate publicity for the Asthmatic Children's Foundation of New York, a residential treatment center in Ossining, New York, for chronically asthmatic youngsters. The children, six to fourteen years old, come mostly from impoverished inner-city neighborhoods in nearby New York City. Their asthma is generally so severe that they can't live at home. Dr. Sanguily's dream is one day to be able to build a swimming pool for them. "I see myself as a kid over and over in the plight of those kids," he says. "I'd love to be able to give them a pool."

Whenever Sanguily spends time with the children in Ossining, he is inevitably drawn back to his own childhood in Cuba and the United States and to the tumultuous part asthma played in his early years. "The life expectancy of young asthmatics in Cuba was very poor. And back then, the 1930s, there was no medication for asthma," he says. "They tried everything. As a kid I drank potions made from leaves. My allergies were so bad that I was forced to live in a room that had nothing in it but a bed. And the bed and pillow were covered with a nonporous rubber covering because we had no plastic. That can get pretty uncomfortable in the hot weather."

For a while the young Sanguily went to the beach in Havana each afternoon strictly to breathe in the salt air because his doctors had told him that the iodine in the air would be good for his asthma. There he met a German swim instructor who encouraged him to start taking lessons. Sanguily found that exercise made him feel much better physically and that his asthma was much more manageable.

In the hope that a complete change in climate and locale might improve his asthma, Sanguily's parents sent him at age twelve to the Hackley School, a private boarding school in Tarrytown, New York. While there he began to swim competitively and to play soccer. Over the next five years he gradually learned to live with his asthma and to extend his physical limits. When he returned to Cuba for vacations, he began to receive allergy shots and new medications for asthma that were then appearing on the market. He also devoted much more time to swimming and training, and for the next eight years competed at the world-class level, his efforts culminating in 1958 with his world record in the breaststroke.

Today, Sanguily describes his asthma as "very persistent" rather than "very severe." But, he quickly adds, "My persistent swimming is the thing that's made the difference." He now has tremendous lung capacity, which he attributes in great part to his swimming, and can blow thirteen liters of air into a spirometer, a device that measures lung function. Six liters or so is normally considered very high.

Sanguily complements his swimming with weight lifting and a menu of daily asthma medication, which includes both pills and inhalers. Occasionally, because of his hectic professional schedule, he'll forget to medicate before getting into the pool at lunchtime. "When I do, I feel it right away," he explains, "usually by the third lap or so. But being a doctor and concerned about my asthma, I know enough not to get involved in any heroics. I get out of the pool, use my spray, and wait about ten minutes. By then, everything gets better and I can continue without any problem."

When asked if it bothers him that he must rely on medication in order to exercise, Sanguily dismisses the idea. "I don't even give it a thought. I'm out there exercising my butt off every day and I'd have one hell of a time if I didn't use medication."

In his family practice Dr. Sanguily sees many people with asthma. "The first thing I do with them is try to deal with the control factor," he says. "I try to give them confidence that they can live without being short of breath. People who aren't asthmatic don't realize how tough it is to be short of breath. Many of the asthmatics I see always have this tremendous fear of suffocating. That fear can be very difficult to overcome."

Next, Sanguily works with parents and children on a vigorous program of cleaning up the home, especially the bedroom of the person with asthma. "I tell them to get everything out of the room that isn't absolutely necessary so that as little dust as possible can collect there." He also discusses medication, its side effects, and when it should be taken. (See chapter 9, "Medication.")

"Above all, I encourage my patients to exercise," says Sanguily. "I think this is paramount. I start by telling them to walk—to just get outside the door and start walking around." Sanguily believes that most people don't know the value of walking and need to be told how beneficial it actually is.

Once they're off and walking, Sanguily encourages them to take up his favorite sport, swimming. "Swimming is the best exercise for asthmatics, but very often it's difficult for people to get to a pool," he says. "Then, too, many people don't know how to swim well enough to get some benefit."

If they can't swim, Sanguily recommends that they use a stationary bike, do daily calisthenics, or try low-impact aerobics. "The important thing is that they exercise regularly," he says.

The general public is greatly misinformed about asthma, says Sanguily, who believes that most people picture asthmatics as inactive, wheezing, sickly types who miss many days of school and work because of their asthma. Sanguily has his own ideas: "People with asthma form a special group," he maintains. "We're not run-of-the-mill. We're persistent. We're achievers. We have a burning need to prove to ourselves that we can do anything that we set out to do. I'll say this with absolute sincerity: My asthma has made me the way that I am today and in a very real sense I'm ecstatic about it."

Dr. Joseph Nieder, a Manhattan pediatric psychiatrist, is also ecstatic—but about his running program. A self-described former "asthma cripple" who has had asthma since he was three, Dr. Nieder at forty-nine keeps up with his daily running program because he finds that it makes a dramatic difference in his asthma. "There have been times when I haven't run," admitted the soft-spoken Nieder during a break at an asthma support group meeting he had come to address, "and my asthma gets worse because my whole physical condition seems to get worse."

Nieder, who started to run in 1974 after finding that he had put on weight and couldn't fit into his trousers anymore, finds that running opens his lungs, gets his heart pumping, and makes it easier to bring up the mucus from his lungs. "Running is a great way to get the day started. It helps my asthma, but it also puts me in a good frame of mind, and when I'm in this positive state, my asthma tends to be much better as well."

Nieder, like many other people with asthma, finds that exercise is a great victory that is relived day after day. "I'm aware that I've run and that once again I've overcome my asthma," he said. "When I look around and see friends who are overweight and who smoke, I feel a great inner sense of victory to have been able to keep running years after my 'healthy friends,' who don't have any medical problems, have stopped exercising." Nieder has run in both the Boston and the New York City marathons and would eventually like to move up in distance and try an ultrarace in the near future, a race longer than twenty-six miles.

"Exercise is healthful. It's beneficial for everyone, even if you do get some asthma every now and then," said Nieder, who always runs with an inhaler clenched in his hand. "The overall effect in terms of life-style, in terms of how you feel about yourself and your asthma, is so far superior if you're able to exercise. Exercise keeps you active, it tones your muscles, and it gets you out of the house. I couldn't be happier."

Francois Haas, Ph.D., the director of the Pulmonary Function Laboratory at the New York University School of Medicine, has for several years been inviting a group of people to come and exercise in a lab three times a week for an hour at a time. The lab, a large, cool room about the size of a basketball half-court, is filled with exercise machines, computers, and technical analyzing equipment. Haas, who has a mild form of exercise-induced bronchospasm himself, is conducting a long-term study to see what effects aerobic exercise has on asthma.

Thus far in the course of his work, Dr. Haas has seen that exercise can help improve lung function. In one study of exercisers with exercise-induced bronchospasm (EIB), he found that the lung capacity of several test subjects starting out on an exercise program dropped 30 percent immediately following exercise. However, after three months of regular lab workouts, their lung capacity dropped only 10 percent following a similar workout.

"It seems that exercise is a form of adaptation, perhaps causing a decreased sensitivity of the airways," explains Haas. "I postulate that the more you exercise, the more you decrease airway sensitivity.

"Theoretically if we take a nonexercising person with asthma and run him on a treadmill at six miles per hour at a heart rate of a hundred and seventy beats per minute, then when he stops he should have asthma. But if you took that same person and trained him over a period of time, his body would become stronger and adapt to the particular stresses of exercise, possibly even showing a decrease in airway sensitivity as well.

"Over time," says Haas, "a run at six miles per hour on the treadmill may only cause the heart to beat a hundred and fifty beats per minute, and while the ventilation before training may have been sixty liters, now that the person is in better aerobic condition, it may be forty-five liters. What we should see as the person works out is that the stimulus for an asthma attack has been reduced, that it takes much more of something to bring on the asthma."

While Haas's scientific research hasn't yet broadened to investigate whether the positive effects of exercise on airway stimulation have any carryover to other asthma triggers, many of his test subjects have found that exercise not only improves their asthma but enables them to be more active.

A good case in point is Sandy Samberg. For most of her life, thirty-nine-year-old Samberg, a physical therapist at New York University Medical Center in New York City, regarded herself as a klutz whenever it came to sports or exercise. "I can remember as a kid wanting to take part in sports and gym class," she says, "but I never did because I didn't think I was made for it. I just couldn't handle any kind of physical exertion. After a couple of minutes, I'd start having these terrible coughing fits and begin gasping for air—even sometimes when I was dancing. Looking back now I realize that it was the asthma, but as I was growing up that just never occurred to me. I just figured that when it came to sports or the physical life, I was like the person who wanted to sing but just couldn't carry a tune. After a while I simply gave up. I didn't bother trying anymore."

Even as an adult, Samberg always turned down invitations to go on skiing trips or vacations to tennis camps. "I used to think, What, me? You've gotta be kidding! I can't run half a block to catch the bus without practically dropping dead in the street. Me play tennis? I used to think my friends were so athletic. I spent a lot of time envying them."

Samberg's life changed once she began exercising. Now all her friends tell her that she can run rings around them. "It's true," she says. "I know I'm in much better shape than they are. Now when I go on vacation, I actually look for something that I know will involve a good deal of physical activity."

Ironically, it was not until she was finally diagnosed as having asthma that Samberg took up running and exercising and, in effect, turned her life around. "The funny thing is," she says, "if I hadn't been diagnosed, I don't think I ever would have started exercising. I'd probably still have the same old opinion of myself—this sedentary person who just wasn't cut out for sports."

In early 1985, Samberg came down with a bad cold that developed into bronchitis. One morning while attending a doctors' meeting at the hospital where she works, she began coughing uncontrollably and gasping for breath. One of the doctors had her taken to the clinic, where she was given standard pulmonary-function tests. It was soon determined that she had asthma, which in this instance had been triggered by her cold but was often triggered by exercising.

Samberg had never had allergies, as did her two brothers, but she considers this a mixed blessing. She now feels that if she had had allergies as a youngster, her asthma would have been detected then. Instead, she had to wait until she was nearly thirty-five years old.

Shortly after being diagnosed, Samberg began taking part in Dr. Haas's exercise project. At first, she was skeptical. "When I started I couldn't even run a quarter mile," she explains, while zipping back and forth on a ski simulator in Haas's lab. "I used to hack and be out of breath, and was weak and tired all the time. I remember saying, 'God, this isn't for me. I can't do this.' But before I knew it I was up to a half mile on the treadmill and later a full mile. I could see changes almost every day."

Initially, Samberg attended Haas's program three times a week at her own convenience. Each session consisted of running on the treadmill while breathing room air, warm air, and cold air (the warm and cold air were administered through a mask). The workouts lasted twenty to thirty minutes. In the beginning, Samberg would experience asthma symptoms after just five minutes of running. Gradually, this stretched to fifteen, then twenty and thirty minutes. At the end of three months, her coughing and fatigue had all but disappeared and she found her confidence growing as her distances and times improved. Today, she no longer experiences any symptoms when she exercises and considers herself asthma-free, although an episode can still be brought on by a bad cold.

Samberg now runs five times a week in the late afternoon, putting in three to five miles each day. She has no difficulty doing eight- or eight-and-a-half-minute miles and has gone as low as seven and a half minutes a mile. She competes regularly in 10-kilometer road races and, should she ever find enough time to train properly, would like to try a marathon. In addition to running, she also works out daily on a stationary bike and does four miles on a cross-country ski simulator.

Samberg says her new life has completely changed her idea of herself. "I don't see myself as sitting on the sidelines anymore, watching other people do things. I certainly don't regard myself as a great athlete, but I do know that I've become someone who's capable of exercising and participating in sports. And that's given me a real sense of accomplishment. I'm in better condition than I've ever been in before, I'm healthier, and I have more energy."

WHAT IS ASTHMA?

An asthma episode is often characterized by difficulty in breathing, prolonged or uncontrollable coughing, wheezing, a tightening of the chest, and increased mucus secretion. Asthma narrows and blocks the airways. It can strike at any age in varying degrees of severity. Episodes can be as brief as a few minutes or can last for hours, even days or weeks, unless properly treated and controlled with medication. To date there are no known cures for the disorder, but with new medications and techniques it can be managed to the point that the person with asthma experiences few or no symptoms or complications.

During an asthma episode, the breathing passages are narrowed in three ways: the muscles surrounding the bronchial tubes constrict, the lining of the tubes (mucosa) swells (much like the area surrounding a splinter in your finger that isn't promptly removed), and there is increased mucus secretion. In all instances, breathing becomes very difficult.

There are many top athletes who refuse to be slowed down by this condition. By receiving proper medical attention they are successfully able to exercise, practice, and compete in their favorite sports. Of course, it took some time to reach the level where they

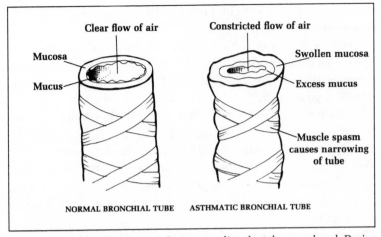

In a normal bronchial tube, muscles surrounding the tube are relaxed. During an asthma episode, the tubes swell, the muscles tighten, and excess mucus is secreted.

were able to manage their asthma. Many uncertainties, and fear in some cases, first had to be overcome as they began to learn about their asthma, what particular triggers set it off, and when medication was needed.

Asthma has a fairly precise medical definition: It is a "reversible obstructive airway disorder." When you read the definition, it sounds so clinical, so removed from the experience of being unable to breathe. But ask a top athlete about his or her asthma and you'll quickly get a vivid image of asthma's scope and the effect it can have on people's lives.

People often have set ideas about world-class athletes, that they never have to go through what the typical person has to deal with, whether it's a bad practice, the urge to quit, or asthma. But this is far from the truth. It doesn't matter if a person is just starting to exercise or has a world record to his or her name, for the problems posed by asthma are just as real for the Olympian as they are for the weekend athlete. "You feel like your lungs are on fire. You feel like they're bleeding. It just hurts too much to breathe," says Bill Koch of his asthma. Koch, the 1976 Olympic 30-kilometer Nordic ski silver medalist, is the best cross-country skier this country has ever produced.

"Asthma is a lot of panic," says Christine Dakin of New York, a principal dancer with the Martha Graham Dance Company whose asthma is triggered by colds. "It's terrifying when you can't get the air out of your chest."

For Dr. Jim Angel, head of the Department of Health and Physical Education at Samford University in Birmingham, Alabama, the thought of asthma makes him flash to a particularly extreme episode he once had. "I thought I would die, it was so bad," says Angel. "I started turning gray, so I went over to an air-conditioning vent in the room and tried to suck the air out of it in order to get myself to breathe."

Many athletes like myself grew up with asthma and for a long time never knew how it felt not to be constantly coughing or gasping for air. Tracy Sundlund, the youngest track coach in Olympic history, has allergenic asthma. "One day when I was ten years old, I went to the doctor's office for my regular appointment," recalls Sundlund, "and he asked me to breathe in deeply. I sucked the air all in through my mouth and then blew it out again. The doctor then said, 'Now breathe in through your nose.' "

Sundlund looked at the doctor as if he were crazy, because with his asthma and allergies he had never really breathed through his nose before. "I had no idea that you did such a thing. 'Why should I do that?' I remember saying. 'The mouth is so much bigger.' "

Asthma is a chronic disease of the air passages that affects approximately 10 million Americans. It's believed that many millions more have undetected asthma and therefore go untreated. Some people who grew up with asthma have an incredibly high tolerance for bronchospasms and just put up with it without really knowing what it feels like to take an easy, deep breath. Others with asthma often neglect seeking professional help, and rely instead on various over-the-counter adrenalinelike medications.

In extreme cases, some people rush to hospital emergency rooms, where their breathing is often stabilized with medications such as adrenaline that can have serious side effects, including rapid heart rate, nausea, and headaches, sometimes migraines. Those who don't control their asthma with proper medical care after such visits return repeatedly to the hospital with each new life-threatening episode.

Tracy Sundlund used to go to emergency rooms frequently for his acute asthma episodes. He recalls traveling to San Diego with his San Luis Obispo, California, club track team for the 1973 state championships. "We stayed at a motel and every night after I had put them all to bed, I'd go off to the local hospital emergency room to get adrenaline shots just so I could breathe and get through the next day.

"Driving back to the motel from the hospital, I could hear my heart pounding in my ears going like a bass drum. It was one great high, but I soon realized that this wasn't the way you're supposed to live."

A short while later, Sundlund began a more realistic and sensible regimen of asthma management that included checking regularly with his physician and taking prescribed medication.

Among children, boys more often than girls have asthma. Asthma tends to run in families that have a history of allergies, hay fever, and asthma. Most of the athletes interviewed for this book have a positive family history for asthma. Generally, when diagnosed and treated in infancy, the asthma shows some signs of improvement by the time the child reaches six years of age. Of the estimated three million children with asthma, it's believed that almost half will lose their "hyperreactive airways"—that is, overly sensitive bronchial tubes—as they move into puberty.

While asthma episodes seem to disappear for most after puberty, medical researchers point out that asthma is most likely only in remission and can flare up again many years later, even in more severe form. Most adults who had asthma in their youth may experience periodic asthma under specific circumstances.

THE BREATHING PROCESS

With each breath, fresh air passes in through the nose and mouth, down through the trachea, or windpipe, and into the large bronchial tubes, one for each lung.

Think of each of your two bronchial tubes as the upside-down trunks of large trees. At the end of each bronchiole (the smaller air tubes, or "branches" of the tree, which sprout off from the main bronchial tubes) are elasticlike air sacs like balloons called alveoli (leaves of the tree), which expand to take in the fresh oxygen and contract to release it. Surrounding the alveoli are small blood vessels, which receive oxygen from the alveoli and then release carbon dioxide to be exhaled.

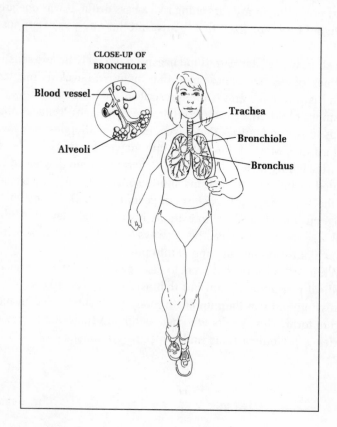

Within the bronchial tubes are small hairlike projections called cilia, which help transport dust, pollen, and other irritants out of the lungs when you cough.

AN ASTHMA EPISODE

Asthma can be brought on by such things as smoke, pollen, food, animal dander, change in weather, excitement, or exercise. Several things happen during a flare-up: In its first, or early, phase the muscles surrounding the bronchial tubes constrict and go into spasm. In the secondary, or late, phase the bronchial tissue becomes inflamed and begins to swell; mucus begins to clog the bronchial tubes, which makes you cough. Once the lining becomes inflamed, the lungs are said to be "twitchy," or more reactive to a trigger, which then makes further asthma episodes more likely.

The end result of the two phases is difficulty in breathing. In the extreme, the person who is not treated after having an acute asthma episode can die from lack of oxygen.

One consistent factor in all asthma episodes, whether or not they are due to allergies, is the hyperreactive (easily irritated), "twitchy" response of the bronchial tubes. Surrounding each bronchial tube is muscle that constricts and dilates by an uncontrolled reflex similar to the involuntary blinking motion of the eyes. In a nonsymptomatic person (someone without asthma), the bronchial tubes constrict naturally in the presence of irritants such as cigarette smoke, air pollution, and some perfumes, for example. However, for a person with asthma, the muscles surrounding the bronchial tubes overreact to the presence of such triggers and other irritants. During this hyperreactive response, the muscles surrounding the bronchial tubes constrict (bronchospasm), the membranes lining the bronchial tubes become swollen and inflamed, and excessive mucus is produced.

In the modern treatment of asthma, it's important to address both stages of asthma before beginning an exercise program: the dilation of the bronchial tubes (the early phase) and the inflamed airways (the late phase). If left untreated, the airways can continue to react long after the initial asthma flare-up, which may result in a more severe episode hours, even days, later.

Many athletes can handle the bronchospasms while they exercise but have difficulty later with a flare-up that occurs in the middle of the night. Often these episodes are more severe than the ones they had while exercising. It's been my experience that the more secondary phases you experience, the more likely you are to become sick, be absent from school or work, and require stronger medications. Therefore, preventing these initial "little exercise episodes" can often keep the more serious asthma from developing.

ASTHMA TRIGGERS

Many things can trigger an asthma episode. Each person's lungs have their own "fingerprint," a unique list of triggers that can contribute to an asthma episode. While a particular trigger may be harmless to one person with asthma, it can lead to a severe episode in another. Proper treatment, therefore, necessitates discovering a person's asthma triggers.

The most common triggers include colds, viral respiratory infections, clogged sinuses; allergens such as animal dander, pollen, house dust, cigarette smoke, perfume, and air pollution; changes in weather and temperature; exercise; sulfites and other food additives; and aspirin. Emotional responses such as laughing, crying, or yelling can also trigger asthma episodes. For more detailed information about asthma triggers, see chapter 5.

WHO NEEDS TREATMENT?

Anyone who has asthma, no matter how mild it seems, should be examined and treated by an allergy and asthma specialist. It's important not to ignore asthma. Asthma doesn't go away by itself, and if left untreated, it can become a serious health risk. Even if you feel that you can handle some mild wheezing and don't think that you need medication, you should still consult with your physician periodically to make certain that your asthma tolerance hasn't become so high that you can no longer differentiate between a mild episode and a serious case.

I've had children who were about to participate in my aerobics program swear to me that their breathing was fine even though I could see that the skin at the base of their throats and collarbones was retracting, a sure sign of severe asthma. The children were not being dishonest, they were just accustomed to quite a bit of asthma. While their asthma might be classified clinically as severe, to them it was nothing to be concerned about because they had learned to live with it. But they were experiencing life from the sidelines— they were generally listless and inactive.

To avoid such a situation, I recommend the use of a peak-flow meter on a regular basis (see chapter 8) in order to get a more accurate picture of your asthma symptoms. The major benefit of the monitor is that it educates you about your asthma by allowing you to connect the feelings you have in your lungs and chest with a quantifiable measurement of airflow. This measurement can often alert you to impending asthma, giving you time to begin proper remedial action before serious asthma symptoms set in. It can also teach you how better to assess your asthma in the future without using a meter.

What is needed for the successful treatment of asthma, according to Dr. William J. Davis, a pediatrician and asthma specialist at Columbia University College of Physicians and Surgeons in New York City, is a comprehensive management plan drawn up between the patient and his or her asthma specialist, making sure that it includes plenty of PET, an acronym for prevention, education, and therapy.

Dr. Davis's three-point plan is summarized as follows:

Prevention: Patients have to recognize and then avoid their asthma triggers. They have to develop the ability to detect asthma problems early on.

Education: Educate the child patient and the parents, or the adult patient and the family, to the full scope of asthma and its treatment. Your physician should keep up with the latest medical advances, and together with the patient and family, develop a plan for managing asthma that should include: (a) when to increase medication, (b) when it's okay to exercise and when you should refrain, and (c) when to call your asthma doctor.

People with asthma should also learn how to use a peak-flow meter in order to get an accurate picture of how much asthma is present.

Therapy: A preventive program for maximum control of symptoms should be developed by the physician and patient with an emphasis on using a minimum of the safest medications with the least amount of side effects. Finding your proper mixture of medication is like getting a pair of eyeglasses with the correct prescription. There is no such thing as "one prescription fits all." Just because you may be uncomfortable with your first prescription, don't give up. You need to communicate fully with your physician about what kind of life you want to lead, what medication works and what doesn't. Don't be surprised by possible side effects of some of the medicines; in time, you can often adjust to them quite well.

FORMS OF TREATMENT

The most common and effective form of asthma control is medication. These medicines fall into five basic groups: beta-adrenergic bronchodilators, cromolyn sodium, corticosteroids, theophylline, and anticholinergics. For a full description of these medications, see chapter 9.

It's not uncommon for a person to avoid taking medication of any sort; I never liked taking even an aspirin. However, when I was finally diagnosed as having asthma and began taking my medication, the benefits were obvious immediately. Other athletes have similar stories. "My asthma doesn't scare me anymore," says Rob Muzzio, the 1987 NCAA national decathlon champion from George Mason University in Virginia and a 1984 Olympic team member.

Muzzio's asthma is triggered by dust and pollen, and in order to train and compete he follows a rigid medication schedule. Every morning he gets up at five o'clock, takes his medication, and then goes back to sleep. He also takes medication again at lunchtime and before going to bed. "Asthma is something that I just had to learn how to deal with and handle," he says. "Without my medication I wouldn't be able to compete."

FIND A GOOD DOCTOR

If you exercise or participate in sports or now wish to begin doing so, then it's very important that you find a physician who not only specializes in asthma and allergies but is also sympathetic to your needs and will help you achieve the quality of life you desire.

Cheryl Durstein-Decker, a champion triathlete from Atlanta, deliberately sought out doctors she knew would be able to help her keep up with the rigorous demands on a three-sport athlete who competes in races 140 miles long. Durstein-Decker recommends that you actively seek a physician who can help: "If your current doctor isn't helping you lead the active life-style that you want, then find another doctor. They are definitely out there. You just have to be persistent in your search."

One of the ways to find a physician who understands the benefits of exercise is to go to a local sports-medicine clinic and get a recommendation from physicians there. (See also chapter 8, "Doctors.")

CONFRONTING YOUR ASTHMA

Asthma shouldn't become the focal point of your life. George Murray, an extraordinary Florida wheelchair athlete and a three-time winner of the Boston Marathon, puts the matter in perspective. "I don't try to analyze my asthma too much," he says. "That's really a difficult and thankless type of endeavor. I've accepted the fact that I'm an asthmatic and that there's no cure for it. If I maintain my medication and I exercise regularly, I'll live the best way that I can. I refuse to make dealing with my asthma my major hobby in life."

Many top athletes speak about "control" whenever they mention their asthma. For them, taking control of their lives means first taking control of their asthma. "If I don't control my asthma, then it's going to control me," says Cheryl Durstein-Decker. "If you can always feel that you're the one who's in control because you know your medication, you know your regimen, and you know how to properly deal with your problem, then there's no reason why you can't push yourself all the way in sports, exercise, and every other area of your life."

When Dr. Jim Angel was diagnosed as having asthma, he initially stopped all exercising, perceiving himself as an "asthma cripple." "After college I had let my physical conditioning lapse," he says. "I told myself, 'I have asthma and I can't do any exercise.' I believed it, too. Then a professor in graduate school told me to start working out and to let my asthma dictate the extent of what I could do. I really needed that kick in the pants to get started. Today my asthma is under control ninety-nine percent of the time. I can do anything I want except for prolonged anaerobic activity, but everything else is fine."

The list of athletes who've taken control of their asthma so they can live more complete and rewarding lives goes on and on. Perhaps the best advice on the subject, however, comes from George Murray, the wheelchair athlete. "Asthma doesn't have to be a big deal," he says. "It doesn't have to affect the quality of your life. Whatever you do, even though you have a medical condition, don't start acting like a patient. Be educated, be smart about your asthma, but don't make asthma out to be more of a pain in the butt than what it needs to be."

COMMON ASTHMA MYTHS

The condition described as "asthma" has been around since earliest times, lending itself to many myths. These myths sometimes keep people from seeking effective medical treatment for their asthma.

Modern medicine is able to stabilize even severe cases of asthma, but if people don't search out the right physician and take responsibility for controlling their asthma, they're not going to benefit from the latest advances in asthma treatment. I once heard about a young Ecuadorean boy who had a mild case of asthma. Perplexed about what to do, his parents bypassed their local doctor and instead consulted a *brujo*, or witch doctor. Closely following his instructions, the parents captured an armadillo and killed it, cooked it, and made their six-year-old son eat the meat. Within a matter of days, the boy was free of all asthma symptoms and supposedly hasn't been bothered since.

While this story comes from a remote region in South America, far from access to modern asthma treatments, there are many people in this country too who think that similar, questionable methods can help relieve or actually cure asthma. Other asthma "cures" I've heard of include fasting for up to six days at a time, eating nothing but parsley juice and cucumbers, and wearing copper-treated heel lifts and shoe inserts. During a call-in radio show in West Virginia a male caller informed me that an enema would get rid of all the poisons in a person's system, asthma included.

There are no miracle cures or secret medical techniques for asthma, so don't go off to Texas or Ecuador in search of armadillos, and don't take an enema and think it will help improve your breathing. Over the years, the medical profession has developed scientifically sound methods for diagnosing, treating, and controlling asthma. These include taking a detailed personal history, performing a physical exam, administering allergy tests when needed, prescribing medication, avoiding allergens, and where possible, making necessary life-style changes. The medications that your doctor prescribes for your asthma have all undergone rigorous, well-designed trials that have proved their usefulness and safety.

Once a person with asthma, or the parent of a child with asthma, fully understands its broad scope and learns what is needed to bring the condition under control, he or she can begin to live a relatively symptom-free life that isn't focused exclusively on dealing with asthma.

One way to reduce dramatically the number of visits to the hospital emergency room and to lower the number of deaths due to asthma is first to clear away some of the misconceptions surrounding asthma. Here are some facts about some of the more common and still prevalent myths.

Myth 1: Asthma is caused by psychological factors.

Fact: Untrue. This is probably the most damaging of all the myths. Asthma is not a psychological illness. In all cases, asthma begins with a physical disorder in the lungs, not with an emotion such as sorrow, anger, or laughter. Strong emotions can, in fact, trigger an asthmatic episode. Just as running around the block elevates pulse and blood pressure temporarily and can bring on asthma, so can an emotion such as sorrow affect a person's already hyperreactive airways. Still, the emotion itself is not the *cause* of asthma, but rather is just a trigger.

It's important to make this distinction between trigger and cause. Confusing the two can very often lead to a delay in treatment and possibly cause a bad medical situation to get much worse. This misguided thinking can also lead you to believe that somehow you brought the asthma on yourself.

Virginia Gilder, a member of the United States women's rowing team, which won a silver medal in the 1984 Olympics, recalls that when she was a child, her father used to tell her that her asthma bouts were caused by her emotions. "He would tell me to pretend that it's not there. As a result I became convinced I could somehow control my asthma by myself. Of course, I couldn't. Even though I was going to an allergist to control the principal symptoms, everyone in my family thought my asthma was psychosomatic. It was a very conflicting situation for me."

Myth 2: Children outgrow their asthma.

Fact: To date, there is not much conclusive medical evidence to support this claim, even though for many children asthma symptoms do become less severe over time and, for many others, seem to disappear entirely. Greg Louganis, the Olympic diver, and Sam Perkins, a former basketball All-American at the University of North Carolina, both had asthma as children but later outgrew it.

Louganis's asthma lasted from birth until he was eight years old; now he merely has hay fever. Early on, Greg's mother was advised by his pediatrician to get her son involved in athletics in order to help increase his lung capacity. With that in mind, she enrolled Greg in tap dancing and acrobatic classes when he was six years old. Eventually, his asthma disappeared and Louganis went on from acrobatics to springboard and platform diving and to a record four Olympic gold medals, two each at the Games in Los Angeles and Seoul. Louganis has now earned the title "The World's Greatest Diver."

Sam Perkins, now the best front-court defender with the NBA Dallas Mavericks, first developed asthma at the age of seven, when he regularly found himself coughing and gasping for breath every time he went out to play. He was diagnosed as having EIB and was put on medication, which he took twice a day without fail for the next seven years. When he turned fourteen, Sam's asthma vanished just as suddenly and mysteriously as it had come on. "All at once," he says, "I found that I could play harder and run longer distances without getting out of breath. The asthma just didn't affect me anymore like it used to." Perkins has been asthma-free for a decade and hopes to stay that way.

Despite the stories of Louganis and Perkins, medical experts caution that even if the asthma has apparently cleared up, in some cases it may actually be in remission, possibly to return later in life. Such people, doctors say, may also be more prone to bronchitis and rhinitis (inflammation of the nose) as they get older.

Myth 3: Moving to a different part of the country will relieve asthma symptoms.

Fact: Packing up your belongings and heading to a warm, humid region of the country is generally not recommended by medical experts as a way of eliminating your asthma. People whose asthma is triggered by local pollens and molds may be leaving old triggers behind but taking on new ones once they settle somewhere else. While some cities have less of one particular type of irritant, most areas have something that can provoke an allergic reaction.

Michael Secrest is a long-distance professional bicyclist who has competed in several editions of the Race AcrossAmerica (RAAM). His health had always been fine and he was never bothered by allergies in his native state of Michigan. However, after moving to Arizona (for the more favorable year-round training conditions), the thirty-seven-year-old Secrest soon started sneezing on a regular basis. Although bothered and perplexed by this, he didn't give it much thought since he was busy preparing for the 1987 RAAM.

Two days into the June race and leading the field through the mountains in Nevada one cool, clear night, Secrest suddenly started wheezing and gasping for breath. His speed soon dropped from an average of twenty miles per hour to fourteen miles per hour as he struggled to take in air. He had no idea what was happening to him or what he should do about it.

After a while he started coughing up blood and mucus, and his speed dropped further. "I had trained for this race for four years," recalls Secrest. "I had a good chance to win and it now looked like I would have to drop out of the race because I couldn't breathe. It was all so crazy. I pulled over to the side of the road and broke down and cried."

A physician who was with Secrest's support team diagnosed his case as asthma and prescribed both theophylline and an albuterol inhaler. Taking these medications along with his first sleep in the race, Secrest awoke two hours later feeling much better. He continued with the medication, and although he still coughed and hacked and experienced pain in his lungs during the seven days it took to reach Washington, D.C., Secrest was eventually able to hold on and win the race.

To this day Secrest is perplexed about the cause of this sole asthma episode. He still lives in Arizona, but his mysterious sneezing has long since stopped and he hasn't had any recurrences of asthma. "It was the strangest thing," he says. "I still don't have any answers."

To all those people who are contemplating a move in order to escape their allergies and possibly their asthma, resist the idea and stay put. Fight your asthma at home. Medical experts recommend that a person with allergy-induced asthma should do all he or she can to manage his or her asthma at home. There are just too many instances of people with allergic triggers who have packed up their belongings and moved their families to a supposedly allergy-free environment, only to find after some heartbreak (and expense) that such places don't exist.

Myth 4: Asthma can't be life-threatening.

Fact: In 1985 more than three thousand people died from asthma. While pharmaceutical companies have developed stronger, more effective medications with fewer side effects than ever before, and while these medications do indeed work, proper treatment of asthma depends on using them regularly and getting asthma under control. This means that persons with asthma have to learn about their condition thoroughly and take their medication faithfully, even after symptoms have disappeared.

What is required in asthma treatment is a teamwork approach: the asthma patient working in tandem with his physician to ensure effective medication and good health. Delays in seeking proper care, overdependence on one medication, denial of symptoms, or spotty medical treatment can lead in part to what some medical authorities are terming an "asthma crisis" in our country. With proper care, no one should ever die of asthma.

Still, people do die from asthma and sometimes these victims are athletes, who, in every other respect, are fit and healthy individuals.

Erik Exum, a football player at Hope College in Holland, Michigan, and Bobby Williams, a promising hockey player in the Boston Bruin (NHL) organization, both died in 1987 after suffering irreversible asthma episodes. In both cases, neither the parents nor the victims ever thought that asthma was life-threatening.

Louann Exum, Erik's mother, feels that she and her son were never sensitive enough to the potential severity of his condition, even though he had lived nearly all his life with bad allergenic asthma and had been brought to hospital emergency rooms for asthma treatment on at least a dozen occasions between grade school and his death at age twenty. It wasn't until she heard about the death of a youngster from asthma three months before her own son's death that Mrs. Exum first considered it a possibility that asthma could kill. Looking back, she now believes that she and Erik were not as aware as they should have been.

"First," says Mrs. Exum, "I think there was a certain amount of denial built into Erik's support group, because he handled the condition in such an independent and seemingly proficient manner. Second, we had no personal contact or knowledge of anyone who had died from the condition until just a few months before Erik died. Third, I believe our medical advisers, acting to the best of their knowledge, and on Erik's behalf, did not withhold information, but rather minimized the potential danger. In retrospect, I believe their approach was well founded in their understanding of the dynamics of stress as it relates to the disease, and their desire to keep that stress under control."

Erik first developed asthma in the second grade. Despite all of his breathing difficulties, Erik was quite active as a child and especially loved sports, from which Mrs. Exum never held him back. On occasions when his asthma became severe, Mrs. Exum would take Erik to the emergency room of the local hospital, where he would receive a shot of an adrenaline derivative. "At such times," says Mrs. Exum, "I would naturally be worried and upset for my child as any parent would, but I never felt as if I had to rush out the door immediately in order to keep him alive."

In high school, Erik took up football and played hard. Throughout these years he took theophylline and albuterol on a regular basis as prescribed by his doctor. Upon graduation, he entered Hope College, where he continued playing football, becoming a standout on the defensive line. Although Erik's participation in athletics did not include aerobic-type exercise, Mrs. Exum is convinced that sport, exercise, and the active life helped her son's asthma by making him physically stronger and better able to handle any asthma episodes.

Late one night in his sophomore year, Erik died from asthma in the corridor outside his dorm room as his roommates looked on in horror. To this day, Mrs. Exum has no clue as to what might have triggered Erik's fatal episode. The night he died, he showed no indications of distress. The only hint that something might have been wrong came about thirty minutes earlier, when he told a friend that he was going to take a nap because he didn't feel well.

"His mental condition was fine and his grades were good," says Mrs. Exum. "He had just become involved for the first time in a wonderful relationship with a girl. Also, he was doing what he loved most—playing football.

"I do know," she adds, "that football and a positive attitude made his life worth living. He had nineteen happy, wonderful years."

Tom Williams shares many of the same feelings about the death of his son, Bobby. "I assumed like everyone else that asthma wasn't a life-threatening situation. I looked upon it as a nuisance illness more than anything else."

Williams recalls watching a TV talk show shortly after his son's death and hearing a woman say that her doctor had assured her that there was no way a person could die from asthma. Williams says he sat there in disbelief, shouting at the TV screen, "It does happen! It does happen! It happened to my son!"

Bobby Williams, twenty-three years old at the time of his death, lived with asthma all his life, and, according to his father, "probably never realized what it meant to take a free breath." As a youngster Bobby went for allergy testing at the Leahy Clinic in Boston and was found to be allergic to "just about everything." He also had exercise-induced bronchospasm.

One of Bobby's worst asthma episodes occurred during the spring pollen season when he was fifteen. He had stayed home from school that day because his allergies were very bad. Mr. Williams, who was a widower at the time, raising five children on his own, returned home from work in the evening to find Bobby nearly unconscious. He rushed his son to the local hospital, where the boy remained in the intensive care unit for almost a week. Bobby recovered, but every spring for the next four years he made at least one visit to the hospital because of a severe asthma episode triggered by pollen, high temperatures, and humidity.

By the time he was nineteen, Bobby's asthma had settled down a bit. It was also at this time that he began lifting weights. Mr. Williams thinks that the weight-lifting routine was actually good for his son's asthma. "The asthma had been much more acute before he began building himself up," he says. "But once he started lifting and got into a training program, he became much more physically fit and we were able to cut out the visits to the hospital every spring."

By this time, Bobby had also developed into an outstanding college hockey player, following closely in the footsteps of his father, who had won a gold medal in ice hockey at the 1960 Winter Olympic Games in Squaw Valley, California, and later played professionally for sixteen years in the National Hockey League.

In the fall of 1986, Bobby signed a pro contract with the Boston Bruins. He was assigned to Flint, Michigan, in the International League and his coach there, who also had asthma, was very high on Bobby's future. He predicted not just a career in the NHL but possibly even stardom, depending on to what degree his asthma held him back.

When Bobby returned home to Boston after the play-offs he took a summer job with a roofing contractor, hoping that the work would help keep him in shape so he'd be ready for training camp in the fall. On June 1, the third day into a bad heat wave and with the pollen count very high, Bobby suffered an acute asthma episode at the job site and died before an ambulance arrived.

"We had talked that morning at seven o'clock just before he went to work," Mr. Williams recalls. "We were going over the final game of the Stanley Cup play-offs, which we'd watched together the night before. Three hours later I received a phone call from the hospital and they said there was nothing they could do for Bobby. The boy who had been working with Bobby said he called out for his inhaler, but it was too late."

At the time of his death, Bobby Williams wasn't taking any medication. But in case of emergencies he always made sure that he had his inhaler with him at all times. "The doctor told him to use his own judgment," Mr. Williams says. "Bobby never wanted to take the medication unless he absolutely had to. He just didn't like the side effects."

Tom Williams is stunned over his son's death and still searching for answers. "You say to yourself that in this case he obviously should have been using some medication. Yet just a week before he died, I was speaking with his coach at Flint and he said Bobby's asthma was fine. He wasn't having any problem with it at all, he told me. And the coach is an asthmatic as well."

If he were allowed to go back in time to that day in June and change anything at all, Mr. Williams says he would not have let Bobby take the construction job. "It was too risky for him—the heat, the humidity, and pollen combined with all that physical exertion was just too much for him.

"But who ever knew it could kill him? The only thing that would really have made a difference in Bobby's case is having some greater awareness of the dangers of asthma. Somewhere along the line somebody should have pulled us aside and said, 'Hey, this illness can kill you. It can really kill you.' "

Myth 5: Corticosteroids should be avoided in the treatment of asthma.

Fact: Steroidal medications definitely have their place in proper medical care. (See chapter 9.) When other asthma medications can't control a severe asthma condition, oral corticosteroids, man-made drugs that duplicate the work of the body's adrenal glands, are often used for their short-term effect. Steroids are also used in long-term treatment when a person doesn't respond well to aggressive treatment with beta-adrenergic medications, cromolyn, and theophylline.

Corticosteroids should not be confused with anabolic (muscle-building) steroids that are used by some athletes as a way of gaining an unfair advantage in sports. Anabolic steroids reportedly stimulate muscle growth, thereby enhancing an athlete's performance. Corticosteroids, a medicine used for severe asthma, don't promote muscle growth but do help shrink swollen bronchial tube linings. Corticosteroids are often used when a person's asthma is particularly persistent.

Myth 6: Asthma is caused by improper breathing and can be cured by learning to breathe properly.

Fact: Asthma is not caused by improper breathing, nor can it be cured by any special breathing techniques. (See chapter 10, "Breathing Exercises.") During an asthma episode some people may panic as they find their air supply diminishing. As a result, they start to breathe faster and faster. This accelerated breathing increases the amount of moisture that the lungs must evaporate. In most cases, rapid breathing intensifies the asthma.

To make it easier to breathe, many people with asthma use special yoga-style breathing techniques to help slow down and control their breathing pattern. It has been shown that yoga-type breathing exercises can help calm a person who's experiencing an asthma episode, thereby possibly helping reduce its potential severity.

Breathing exercises can play an important part in asthma management but shouldn't be substituted for medication unless under the advice of a physician, because they won't relieve bronchial constriction and tissue inflammation. While breathing exercises may be effective in calming a person, they should serve only as an adjunct to a total asthma management program, not be used in lieu of one.

Myth 7: Over time, asthma will permanently damage the lungs.

Fact: Asthma is defined as a *reversible* obstructive airway disorder. The bronchial tubes are affected adversely during an asthma episode, but these changes are reversible either on their own or with medication, leaving no permanent damage. Only in very severe chronic and rare cases is permanent damage inflicted by asthma. While people may sometimes describe an acute and prolonged asthma episode as one that "burns the lungs," the condition is reversible once the inflammation goes down, although the symptoms may linger for months.

Asthma is sometimes confused with emphysema, a lung disorder that is most often caused by cigarette smoke. Emphysema is an irreversible condition in which the air sacs (alveoli), not the air tubes, are damaged. Asthma does not cause or lead to emphysema or other lung-damaging diseases.

Myth 8: Asthma results in stunted growth.

Fact: Many parents believe that their children will not reach their full size because of asthma and the medication that they take. The vast majority of asthma medication has no ill effects on a child's physical development. In severe cases of asthma, oral corticosteroidal medications must be used over the long term, and while they may interfere with growth patterns, many people can use these drugs for long periods without any adverse effects continuing into adulthood. The good news is that most children with asthma never need such powerful medications and don't exhibit any abnormal growth patterns.

Myth 9: You cannot lead a normal life if you have asthma.

Fact: You can control your asthma instead of letting it control you. In speaking with people with asthma, I've observed that many of them have chosen one of two approaches to dealing with asthma. One is to ignore the asthma, and the other is to live in a sterilized closet. Those who ignore asthma believe that a lot of the problem is in their heads, and that if they were tough, they wouldn't let it affect how they live. This type believes that if they "just don't let it affect me," it will go away. These people spend a lot of time in the emergency room as their method of dealing with asthma.

The second type is terrified of their condition and afraid to include anything in their lives that might trigger an episode of asthma. They start by avoiding simple things, like cigarette smoke and feather pillows, and build upon this list until they avoid most food, neighbors' homes, the outdoors, and anything foreign. They don't just avoid participating in sports; they even avoid watching an exciting match for fear of provoking some asthma.

Both extreme cases inhibit the quality of life possible for asthmatics. In both cases, the asthma is controlling the person, rather than the person controlling the asthma. There is another way.

I like to compare controlling asthma to having clean, healthy teeth. I do several things during the day to make sure that my teeth are clean and well cared for. I see my dentist twice a year, and I go more often if I suspect a problem, like a pain in a particular tooth when I bite down. I try to see my dentist promptly when I'm having trouble, and don't wait until the tooth has rotted before giving him a call. But, do I *think* about having clean teeth? No! These are just things I do automatically as part of my daily routine, not things to focus my attention on. But just because I don't focus much mental energy on them doesn't mean that I don't do what's necessary to have healthy teeth.

It's the same for asthma. At first, using an inhaler and a peak-flow meter, and recording exposures to allergens and performances may sound like a lot of work, but these things will quickly become automatic. You won't give them a second thought once you've made them part of your routine day.

Myth 10: People with asthma can't exercise.

Fact: Absurd! After consulting with their physicians (just like everyone else!), people with asthma have the opportunity to exercise regularly. Of course, they will need to increase their exercise tolerance gradually to enjoy any number of sports.

People with asthma need not lead sheltered lives. You can learn how to control asthma so that you can participate in your favorite sport or exercise routine. In the 1984 Olympic Games, forty-one medals were won by Olympians with asthma. In the 1988 Summer Olympics in Seoul, sixteen medals were won by Olympians with asthma. In spite of their medical condition, these athletes became the best in the world in many different sports.

Who says people with asthma shouldn't exercise? Certainly none of the following medal winners.

The Olympic Games, Los Angeles, 1984: Medals Won by American Athletes with Exercise-Induced Bronchospasm

Total U.S. Olympic team members: 597
Number with asthma: 67
Total number of medals won: 174
Number of medals won by athletes with asthma: 41

Sport	Gold	Silver	Bronze
Basketball	4		
Cycling	3	3	2
Equestrian		1	
Field Hockey			2
Modern Pentathlon		2	
Rowing	1	4	
Shooting		1	
Swimming	5	1	
Track and Field	1	1	
Volleyball		3	
Water Polo		4	
Weight Lifting			1
Wrestling	1		
Yachting		1	
TOTALS	15	21	5

The Olympic Games, Seoul, 1988:
Medals Won by American Athletes with
Exercise-Induced Bronchospasm

Total U.S. Olympic team members: 611
Number with asthma: 53
Total number of medals won: 94
Number of medals won by athletes with asthma: 16

Sport	Gold	Silver	Bronze
Basketball	2	1	
Rowing		2	1
Swimming		2	
Track and Field	2		
Water Polo		4	
Wrestling		1	
Yachting	1		
TOTALS	5	10	1

CASE CLOSED!!!

ASTHMA TRIGGERS: ALLERGIES

Why an asthma episode begins is not yet fully understood by doctors or asthma researchers. It is well known, however, that people with asthma may be affected by different "triggers," factors that bring on an asthmatic episode. Many people with asthma have a fairly good idea of what their particular triggers are and are therefore able to avoid them or control their response to some degree. Other people keep discovering new triggers that affect them. It may be ragweed at a particular season of the year, it may be exercise, it may be a food additive, such as sulfite.

If you have asthma, you need to take the time to identify your specific asthma triggers. Keep a detailed record chart, or diary, noting your symptoms and the duration and intensity of your response after exposure to a suspected trigger. Also note the different side effects after taking your medications.

To facilitate this record keeping, Nancy Sander, the founder of Mothers of Asthmatics (MA), has come up with an excellent record-keeping system called *The Asthma Organizer* ($20, Mothers of Asthmatics, Inc., 10875 Main Street, Suite 210, Fairfax, VA 22030, 703-385-4403) that is packaged in a sturdy three-ring binder. This handy notebook is the perfect tool for keeping track of triggers, medicine, doctor visits, and peak-flow readings, all of which will help in gaining control over asthma.

There are numerous factors that can trigger an asthma episode. Among the most common are:

1. Allergies
2. Food and food additives such as sulfites and tartrazine
3. Aspirin and other medications
4. Emotions
5. Irritants, such as tobacco smoke and fumes from chemical cleaners
6. Weather and climatic conditions, including air pollution
7. Colds and other respiratory infections
8. Exercise

This chapter addresses allergies; the other triggers are discussed in detail in chapters 6 and 7.

ALLERGIES: THE NUMBER-ONE ASTHMA TRIGGER

Approximately thirty-five million Americans have some form of allergy, whether it be to airborne pollens, cold temperature, insect bites, pollutants, dust, food, penicillin, or aspirin. Symptoms can include itchy eyes, a runny or stuffy nose, a sore, scratchy throat, incessant sneezing, hives, swelling, fatigue, and, in the case of people with asthma, wheezing, difficulty in breathing, and mucus buildup in the airways.

Jim Ryun, former world record holder in the mile and 1,500 meters and currently one of the top Masters (the category for runners over forty years of age) mile runners in the world, is asthmatic and severely allergic to pollen and ragweed. Ryun's allergies were first detected in high school when his track coach, Bob Timmons, noticed that his star runner would often finish his workouts looking pale and feeling extremely weak and tired. Timmons sent Ryun to an eye, ear, and nose doctor and finally to an allergist, who gave him allergy tests. He was diagnosed as being oversensitive to various pollens and started on a program of desensitization shots.

Year-round for nearly fifteen years, Ryun received allergy shots twice a week, the dosage varying with the amount and types of pollen in the air. This therapy, supplemented with antihistamines, helped a good deal but was never sufficiently effective to keep the runner symptom-free. Because he was unable to breathe properly, Ryun's training suffered.

Ryun continued to be hampered by allergies and eventually found himself at the mercy of sports reporters and critics, who, after witnessing some of his wildly inconsistent and erratic performances, began suggesting that perhaps he choked in big races and that his troubles were really psychological in nature.

"There's no question that the allergies affected my running performance," Ryun says. "My times would always fall off during pollen season, even in training. People said I had a psychological problem or that I raced too much and was burned out. I never

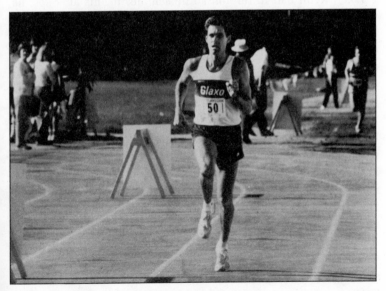

Jim Ryun.

thought so. I'd go for a race in another part of the country where the air quality was different and I'd do fabulously well. It was very frustrating that in the beginning no one clearly understood what was wrong with me, not even me."

Ryun didn't learn until he was well past his prime as a runner that his allergies were part of a larger medical picture that included asthma, both allergenic and exercise-induced. For years, the only solutions available to him had been allergy shots and antihistamines, and without them, he admits, he would never have been able to compete during the pollen and ragweed season. However, in 1984 Ryun was finally diagnosed as having asthma. Since then, he has used only a bronchodilator inhaler to medicate himself and has been amazed by the difference in how he feels and performs on the track.

"What the medication does is let me maintain my conditioning level," says Ryun. "With just the albuterol inhaler I can keep the allergies and the asthma in check without any allergy shots. And the beauty of it is that I no longer have any of the side effects that the antihistamines used to give me."

When Ryun had to rely on antihistamines for his allergies, he would sometimes be so fatigued that even a short run would be tiring. Other times he'd take a pill and not only could he run at top speed, but he felt as if he were flying. "There was always that tremendous variation with antihistamines but not with the inhaler," says Ryun. "It's been wonderful. I only wish that I had known about it sooner."

Airborne pollen from plants, trees, and grasses are the culprits that trigger many asthma episodes. Some areas of the country have much higher pollen levels than others. In 1971, Ryun moved to Eugene, Oregon, to begin preparations for the 1972 Olympic summer games. Eugene is the unofficial running capital of the United States and has been since the 1960s when Bill Bowerman, the renowned long-distance coach, began attracting many of the best American and foreign track athletes to his running program at the University of Oregon. After graduating, many of these athletes stayed on in Eugene to train with Bowerman. Eventually, they came to form a small community whose focus was running.

The National Track and Field Championships have been held in Eugene many times, and in 1984 the city was host to the Olympic track-and-field trials. Eugene is certainly idyllic for runners who don't have allergy or asthma problems. But if you happen to be allergic and/or asthmatic like Jim Ryun, Keith Brantley, John Powell, Doug Padilla, Pat Porter, Karin Smith, and other outstanding track-and-field athletes, Eugene is also the ragweed and ryegrass capital of the country, an area with some of the highest pollen counts ever recorded.

When Jim Ryun moved to Eugene, his allergies had not been troubling him for a while and he was looking forward to living and training in the unique running environment Eugene had spawned. His hopes were dashed almost immediately when he discovered that the high pollen levels prevented him from being able to train. No matter how hard he worked, he was unable to make any progress and constantly felt tired. His performance level declined miserably. After just six months he packed up and relocated to Santa Barbara, California.

According to Keith Brantley, the Athletics Congress 1987 Road Racer of the Year and an asthmatic, the pollen in Eugene is so bad that "some people have to wear surgical masks when they run. You can actually see pollen floating in the air." But like other people with asthma and allergy-prone athletes, Brantley has no choice: If a major race is being held in Eugene, he has to be there to compete.

Brantley and other athletes such as Pat Porter, the seven-time national cross-country champion, try to circumvent the pollen problem by arriving in Eugene at the last minute and using an arsenal of medication. But this doesn't always do the trick. In 1986, at the National Championships, held during the height of the spring pollen season, Brantley found himself unable to breathe while running the 10,000 meters. "All of a sudden it was as if I got hit in the face with a two-by-four," Brantley says. "I couldn't go another foot and had to drop out of the race. It was just too difficult to breathe."

When it comes to allergies, avoidance of the triggers and medical treatment are the best courses of action. It's not recommended that you go to the extreme of putting your home on the market and moving out of town because of high pollen rates. In many cases, even severe allergies can be managed successfully with medication and/or immunotherapy. Still, there may be limits to how hard you can push yourself athletically when your allergies are particularly bothersome.

While tree pollens are a major asthma trigger, there are others that are just as potent. James Wofford and Bruce Davidson are two athletes who encounter a very special problem whenever they are engaged in their sport: Both men are world-renowned equestrians who are allergic to horses.

This inconvenience hasn't held them back, though, and neither has their asthma. Wofford, an Olympian in 1968 (silver team medal), 1972 (silver team medal), and in 1984 in Los Angeles, is highly allergic to a number of things, including dust, cat dander, ragweed, pollens, and "just about anything that grows," he says. It's ironic that Wofford is also allergic to horses, to the animal he spends most of his day with.

"When I'm leaning over a horse's neck," he recalls, "and it's around the middle of April on the first warm, humid day in Virginia when all the grass-pollen air is just starting to really come out, I'm in for trouble. Inhaling the spume off my horse's neck at this time— well, that's usually good for a nice huge asthma attack."

Two to three times a year Wofford has asthma episodes, each one lasting about thirty minutes. None has ever affected his performance in competition because they always come on afterward while he's cooling down, common for some asthmatics. Although he retired from international competition in 1984, Wofford doesn't intend to stop riding. His advice to all those who have asthma and bad allergies but still want to pursue a sport they love is very simple: "Learn how to live with your allergy or asthma and just keep on doing the best that you can."

Bruce Davidson has had allergenic asthma for as long as he can remember. From childhood through adolescence, he received eight allergy shots a week and on numerous occasions had to be taken to hospital emergency rooms after an asthma episode had left him nearly unconscious.

Davidson was on the Olympic equestrian team in 1972, 1976, 1984, and 1988, winning a silver team medal in Munich in 1972 and gold team medals in Montreal in 1976 and Los Angeles in 1984. In 1974 and 1978 he was the world champion in individual competition, the only person in the history of the sport ever to win it twice. He has also been the American champion seven times and currently holds the title. Bruce Davidson has never let his asthma keep him from participating in sports, even going against his parents' orders at times. "As a child, whenever I played baseball or ran around, I was always encouraged to stop and sit down so I wouldn't bring about any health problems," he says. But Davidson wouldn't accept a sedentary life as a solution to asthma.

When his love of horses became a passion, it brought with it more problems with asthma. "I was always told that I never should go into a stable because of all the dust and horse dander," says Davidson. "I was certainly not allowed to ride a horse because that instantly gave me breathing problems." Despite this, Davidson continued to go to the stables and ride. He had to take more medication when he was riding, but it was worth it. "I'd get attacks, but I always kept them to myself because I knew that if my family found

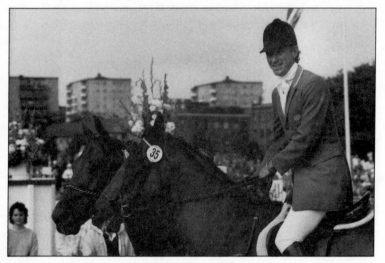

Bruce Davidson.

out they would try to keep me away from the horses. I never told anyone but instead took my atomizer [inhaler] along with me to the stables. Whenever I was out riding, I'd stop every once in a while, hop off my horse, use the medication my doctor gave me, get back on the horse, and keep going."

In addition to riding every day, Davidson goes out for a run five days a week, averaging five to seven miles a workout. His asthma affects him, but he premedicates with an inhaler and again when he's finished. He finds that this carries him through the run with no problems. Davidson has also been teaching riding for some time, and among his students have been several children with serious cases of asthma. He gives them no special treatment and has them training with a peer group of nonasthmatics. If any difficulties develop, the youngsters stop, take their medication, and then continue with their lessons.

"If you have asthma, you have to realize that it can be controlled," says Davidson. "And the first thing you've got to do is get on top of the situation mentally and make up your mind that you're going to deal with it, that you can be as competitive as the next guy. Living with asthma isn't easy. It's not something that you can one day just give away to someone else. But you certainly can find ways to live with it and go on to do whatever you want with your life." I think so, too.

WHAT IS AN ALLERGY?

Take a walk on a balmy day in spring. Flowers are blooming and their perfume fills the air. Trees are coming out of their winter slumber and their bright green leaves add color to the landscape. Close your eyes and take a deep breath. For many, this is as close as they'll come to paradise on earth. Unless, of course, they happen to have allergies.

When a person sensitive to pollen inhales pollen (an allergen) from trees, grass, or flowers, an overreaction to the pollen begins in the nose or bronchial tubes, often triggering an allergic reaction.

You can better understand the allergic process by comparing it to a splinter in your finger. After the tiny splinter goes into the skin, redness appears, there is some swelling, and a certain level of discomfort occurs as the body attempts to fend off the foreign substance.

When you have an allergic reaction to dust, dander, or pollution, the body releases too many histamines and other substances in order to protect itself from what it senses to be a foreign and dangerous substance. In response, the eyes typically become red and itchy. You start to sneeze, and soon your nose gets congested. Just as your finger may be sore until the splinter is removed (and for some time after, as well), your allergy symptoms will persist as long as you're in contact with the offending allergen and for a while after.

Medically, here's what occurs when an allergy-sensitive person comes into contact with an allergen (or antigen): Immunoglobulin E (IgE) allergy antibodies exist in everyone and are found on the outside of *mast cells*. Mast cells are located in the lining of your skin, respiratory tract, and gastrointestinal tract. Inside these cells are histamines. When an allergen such as grass or pollen comes in contact with a specific IgE grass-pollen antibody in the allergic person, the mast cell releases histamines, which act as mediators in a defensive measure to protect the body. It's then that the allergic person starts his or her reaction.

If the mast cells of your skin are affected, raised welts (hives) appear or eczema may develop, causing the skin to redden, itch, swell, blister, and scab. Mast cell overreaction in the digestive area could mean diarrhea or nausea. When eyes, nose, or throat are affected, typical "hay fever" symptoms result: inflammation of the nose (allergic rhinitis is what the allergy doctor will write in his or her notes), sneezing, and itchy red eyes are common symptoms. When the allergic reaction occurs in the lungs, it can bring on classic asthma symptoms: wheezing, a hacking cough, "tightness" in the chest.

Heredity also plays a strong role in allergies. If one of your parents has or had hay fever, you stand a 30 percent chance of de-

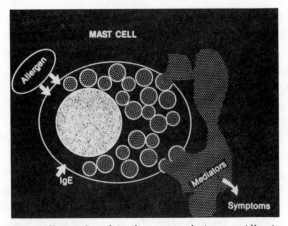

Mast cells are found in the nose and airways. Allergic individuals produce IgE antibodies to specific allergens that rest on the outside of the mast cells. When a person comes into contact with these allergens, they attach to the IgE antibody on the mast cell. Histamines are then produced to combat the allergen, which often then leads to an asthma episode. (*Glaxo*)

veloping it as well. If you have the misfortune of having two parents with hay fever, your chances of developing it shoot up to 70 percent. If either of your parents has asthma, you are at high risk to develop not only asthma but hay fever as well.

CONSULTING AN ALLERGIST

Of the thirty-five million Americans who have allergies, it's estimated that nearly nine million also have asthma. If you believe your asthma is triggered by allergies, it's important to establish exactly what the offending antigens are. This can be done through careful observation and by keeping a daily written diary of your symptoms, their severity, your activities and diet, and weather conditions. Once you have some idea of what may be bothering you, and if the condition warrants medical attention, make an appointment with a board-certified allergist. In all likelihood, he or she will give you a "prick" skin test and/or a RAST (radioallergosorbent test), and/or a multi-test, then prescribe medication and perhaps begin immunotherapy (also known as desensitization shots or "allergy shots") as well.

Testing

During a "prick" skin test, or "scratch" test, several diluted extracts of antigens such as ragweed, tree pollens, or dust are placed on the forearm or back. Then small scratches (one per antigen) are made in the skin to introduce the antigens to the body. If you are allergic to a substance, within twenty minutes a raised welt (hive) will be visible and itchy, indicating that you are allergic to that substance.

In a RAST (radioallergosorbent test), a fairly new alternative to skin testing, one blood sample is taken from the patient and analyzed for specific IgE antibody levels. The benefits of this test are that it's relatively simple, painless, and symptom-free. This is good news for people whose allergies are so extreme that they can't stop taking antihistamines, medications that typically invalidate skin-test results. The limitations of RAST testing are that it's more expensive than skin testing, takes more time to yield results, and, in picking out some rare allergens, is not as effective as skin testing. Many doctors use both tests.

In a multi-test, a small plastic device is placed on the arm, and its small points deliver the allergens to the arm with relatively little pain.

ALLERGY REMEDIES

There are several different approaches to defending against allergy episodes. Some will work better than others, depending on the severity of your case.

Over-the-Counter-Medications: Prior to seeking out an allergist for an examination, many people resort to over-the-counter (OTC) medications for relief of their symptoms. Nonprescription antihistamine medications such as Actifed, Chlor-Trimeton, and Sudafed fill the shelves of local pharmacies and supermarkets.

For temporary relief of symptomatic distress, these medications may be effective, but some people find that they have noticeable side effects, including excitability, drowsiness, and blurred vision. Also, nasal decongestants often constrict the blood vessels of people with hay fever, causing a rebound effect. Once the medication wears off, the symptoms rebound, returning in more severe fashion as even more mucus is secreted in response to an allergen. Because of these inherent problems, many people find OTC medications to be ineffective for treating their long-term allergies. However, if your allergy season lasts for only a week or two, or is relatively mild, then OTC medications may offer adequate relief.

Prescription Medications: For people with hay fever, many allergists now prescribe terfenadine (sold under the trade name Seldane), the most popular antihistamine, which successfully inhibits allergy symptoms in most people without causing drowsiness.

Nasalcrom (for the nose) and Opticrom (for the eyes), two prescription cromolyn sodium medications, are also being successfully employed to prevent allergy episodes from starting. If taken prophylactically before symptoms begin, these drugs can prevent the onset of allergic reactions in about half of the people who take them. Both medications keep the mast cells from releasing histamines during an allergic response.

The particular drawback to these cromolyn medications is that they can't be taken for relief once symptoms have already occurred. They must be taken preventively several times a day and employed over a period of time to be truly effective in allergy relief.

Many physicians also prescribe steroidal nose sprays for allergies. These sprays, such as beclomethasone dipropionate (sold under the trade names Beconase and Vancenase) and beclomethasone dipropionate monohydrate (Beconase AQ and Vancenase AQ), inhibit or reduce mucus production and shrink the swollen, inflamed tissues. These steroidal medications are very effective and have few side effects typical of steroids, since they are taken in spray, not oral, form and so have approximately one-twentieth of the medication in one pill. (See chapter 9, "Medication.") Since inhaled steroidal sprays go directly to the congested airways, they have little effect on the adrenal glands and, hence, virtually none of the side effects of steroids taken orally.

Immunotherapy

Immunotherapy has many different names: hyposensitization, de-sensitization, or, more commonly, "allergy shots." Immunotherapy is not an allergy cure, but it can lessen the need for the long-term use of medication in some people. Although there are many allergists who champion immunotherapy, there are just as many physicians and patients who question its overall effectiveness.

After administering a skin test in order to identify specific allergens, an allergy specialist will often prescribe a course of immunotherapy treatment. No drugs are used in immunotherapy. The basic theory behind the procedure is that after being injected on a weekly basis with low-concentration doses of whatever it is you're allergic to, the IgE levels of that antibody will be lowered and you will then become desensitized to that particular allergen.

If treatment is successful, the next time you come into contact with the allergen—a field of freshly cut grass, for example—you won't get the familiar allergic responses. Immunotherapy appears to work best for persons allergic to pollens and dust.

For immunotherapy to be effective, a long-term commitment is required. Treatments should be continued for three to five years, with allergic symptoms usually subsiding after one to two years. Still, persons who stop taking their weekly injections have a 50 percent chance of relapse.

Immunotherapy is not a cure-all for every person with allergies. However, for persons with asthma who have been found to have only allergy-triggered episodes or have particularly severe allergy-induced episodes, immunotherapy might be the best approach.

Consult your allergist. If he or she can find exactly what you're allergic to, immunotherapy may be beneficial. Prime candidates for immunotherapy are people who are unable to completely avoid their allergens, whose episodes cannot be controlled at all times by medication alone, and whose allergies are present for more than a few weeks during a season. Over a typical three-to-five-year course of immunotherapy treatment, such people can expect a reduction of some sort in the severity of their condition.

Efforts by the American College of Physicians are now under way to ensure that patients are properly diagnosed for allergies. While allergy testing has long been the primary indicator of whether or not someone is allergic, according to allergy expert Dr. Paul P. VanArsdel, Jr., and Dr. Eric P. Larson, authors of the American College's 1989 allergy paper published in *The Annals of Internal Medicine*, doctors should be alerted to the fact that allergy testing should be used only as a tool to help verify a doctor's diagnosis that is already based on (1) the patient's medical history and (2) the patient's symptoms.

When properly used, allergy tests are certainly valuable diagnostic tools, say these two University of Washington Medical School doctors, but no test, they point out, not even an allergy skin test, is good enough to be used as the sole basis for allergy diagnosis. To rely only on skin tests could lead to error in both eventual diagnosis and treatment.

The new guidelines recommended by Drs. VanArsdel and Larson also cover testing procedures. While there are hundreds of allergens that can be used in skin testing that are approved for use by the Food and Drug Administration, it's rarely necessary to use more than fifty different ones on a patient; Dr. VanArsdel usually tests with only twelve to twenty allergens to isolate the source of an allergy. Some other physicians, however, may use as many as three hundred different ones in skin-testing a patient; this is a time-consuming, uncomfortable, expensive, and unnecessary procedure that should be modified.

Reducing Pollen Allergens

For someone who exercises outdoors or spends a good deal of time outside, it's difficult to avoid pollen completely because it's blown around by the wind. The following tips may help you avoid pollen exposure as much as possible.

- Minimize grass allergy in the summer by having your lawn cut. Researchers say that regularly clipping grass to three inches effectively keeps it from blooming and releasing its allergy-aggravating spores.
- While it's better to have someone else cut the grass for you, if you do it yourself wear a mask that will cover both your mouth and your nose. Don't reuse this mask.
- Avoid strenuous exercise when pollen levels are highest. In rural areas, pollen levels are highest at 3:00 P.M. because the temperature is generally high, the humidity low, and the wind usually blows strongest at this time. In large metropolitan areas, pollen levels are generally highest around 7:00 P.M. The heat generated by people and buildings during the day keeps the pollen high in the air, but it starts to descend in the cool of the evening.
- Try to avoid areas such as construction sites or farms, where the air may have a higher accumulation of dust and pollen.
- Air conditioners in cars can often trigger an allergic reaction because they harbor both pollens and molds. Before entering your car, close the air vents, open the windows, and turn on the air conditioner. After several minutes, molds and spores should be dispersed from the air conditioner and it will again be safe to use.
- Keep windows closed during the pollen season.
- Use an air conditioner during pollen season and make sure it's switched to "Recycle." Clean or change your air filter regularly.
- Equip your heating system with a dust-filtering device or install an electrostatic air cleaner to filter air in your home.

- If you have experienced a very strong allergic reaction while outdoors, your skin, hair, and clothing will most likely still contain remnants of the allergens. Take a shower as soon as possible to rinse the pollen off your body. Shampoo your hair and change your clothing as well. If you wear contact lenses, rinse them off with cleaning solution.

Allergy-Proofing Your Home

For some people with allergies and asthma, symptoms may warrant a complete overhaul of their home. Allergens are plentiful outdoors and can be difficult to combat. In your own home you have more control over what enters the house and therefore a better chance of breathing comfortably during your particular allergy season. Some children find that thoroughly cleaning the house makes it dust-free and keeps them out of the hospital. The mother of Rick DeMont (the swimmer who had his 1972 gold medal wrongfully stripped from him because he was taking an asthma medication that contained epinephrine) took out his rug and mopped his bedroom every day.

The basic practical strategy in keeping a home as allergen-free as possible is to mount a room-to-room search. The following tips are helpful:

- If you have wallpaper, check to see if there is any mold growing on it or underneath any tiny flaps or places where the seams of the paper meet. You can remove mold using a solution of vinegar and water.
- If you have wall-to-wall carpeting, shag rugs, and/or upholstered furniture, either get rid of them or at the very least keep them out of your bedroom. These items are great traps for dust and pollen.
- Drapery is another big dust and pollen collector. Avoid venetian blinds, which collect dust and are difficult to clean. Roll-down window shades are preferable.
- Avoid doing housecleaning, or else wear a mask while cleaning. When dusting, use a damp cloth to remove dust. A dry

dust mop has a tendency to spread the dust around the room.

- When cleaning, avoid using ammonia or pine oil, two substances that are common inhaled antigens. Acceptable substitutes include vinegar, soap, chlorine bleach, and baking soda.
- Keep the bedroom door closed, especially when sleeping.
- Remove all book collections from bedrooms. They are great dust collectors. Also, check the TV, stereo, and other electronic appliances for dust.
- Keep the bedroom as free of clutter as possible.
- Make sure your air-conditioner filter is changed regularly and that the switch is turned to the "Recirculate" or "Recycle" setting. Air conditioners are great pollen traps. Dirty ACs can harbor different types of molds in their dark and damp recesses. Clean them regularly.

You can take these precautions too far, as Dr. Joe Nieder, the Manhattan child psychiatrist, found out. Nieder, whose asthma is triggered by pollen, can laugh about it now, but several years ago he took his housecleaning to the furthest extreme.

"I took out all the drapes and venetian blinds from every room and had every piece of furniture in the apartment covered with plastic," says Nieder, who admits that these measures were in vain and that his asthma didn't improve as he had hoped.

"I mistakenly believed that if I could avoid all triggers in my home—what I really wanted was to live in a glass bubble—that I wouldn't have asthma anymore," he says.

It didn't work out as Nieder had expected. "The apartment was bare and sterile and my wife was ready to leave me," he says. "So I had everything changed back. I still have asthma, but I found out the hard way that you can't go to such extremes in trying to cope with it."

6

OTHER ASTHMA TRIGGERS

FOOD ALLERGIES AND INTOLERANCES

Active people enjoy eating; when I was in the midst of training, my mother used to say that I ate like a family of four. Unfortunately, those few who have food allergies and intolerances must constantly exercise caution and restraint in their diet. This is doubly true for people with asthma, since an adverse reaction to a particular food could lead to an asthma episode.

Allergists and medical researchers distinguish between a food allergy and a food intolerance. Strictly speaking, an individual is said to be "allergic" to a food only if specific IgE antibodies to that food (allergen) are present on the outside wall of the mast cells (see chapter 5). If there are no IgE antibodies, then the person has what is known as an "intolerance" to the food.

In practical terms, it makes little difference whether one is allergic or intolerant to a particular food, since both conditions can produce the same symptoms. What is important is to learn which foods you're sensitive to and to avoid them as much as possible.

Food Challenges

If you suspect that you have a food allergy or intolerance, it's best verified in a physician's office in carefully monitored test-by-test double-blind food challenges. *Double-blind* means that neither the doctor nor the patient is aware which food is in the capsule the patient has to swallow.

After you take a capsule, your doctor will note your reaction, if any, and go on to the next capsule. Most doctors report that double-blind studies often show that people are, in fact, not that sensitive to a food. Most children suspected of being sensitive to sugar intake by their parents, teachers, and friends, come up negative when tested.

If at any point you demonstrate a severe reaction, your doctor will recommend that you avoid that particular food or substance in the future. Only when you have said good-bye to the food and have successfully eliminated if from your diet can you be assured that you will be symptom-free.

It's important to note that children who are told by their doctor and parents that they have to avoid eating chocolate, cakes, nuts, bread, or sugars often begin to think that they're different from other children or that something about them is odd. Great care must be taken to make children understand why a particular food has to be avoided and that they are not different from any of their friends. Also, if your child's intake from a particular food group has to be limited, be sure to consult with your doctor about substitute foods of similar nutrient content, especially for milk, whose calcium children need for strong growing bones.

For many people, sensitivity to food doesn't manifest itself so much in the obvious allergic reactions as in a number of subtle yet nagging symptoms that persist from day to day. These can include fatigue, moodiness, muscle aches and pains, and difficulty in carrying out a sustained bout of physical exercise. The medical profession is divided on whether or not these symptoms can be entirely ascribed to food allergies and intolerances. While there is no scientific data to support such claims, some athletes do find relief by undergoing an exhaustive series of tests and then eliminating specific foods from their diet.

If you choose to explore this route, make sure that the foods you eliminate are replaced by foods with equivalent nutrients, so your new diet is nutritionally sound.

Food allergies and intolerance are rare, and discovering which items give you trouble can become quite tricky. Many times the offending agent isn't the food itself but what's been put into it before it reaches your table. These additives can include sulfites (used as preservatives), food colorings (especially tartrazine), flavor-enhancing chemicals like the MSG commonly found in Chinese cuisine, contaminants such as insecticides (sprayed on fruits and vegetables), and antibiotics and hormones (found in meat and poultry products).

When persons with a food allergy or intolerance consume something they are sensitive to—eggs, dairy products, pecans, and shell-fish are the chief offenders—they may develop one or more of the classic allergy symptoms: hives, itching, sneezing, wheezing, diarrhea, and/or vomiting. In certain severe cases they may also have an anaphylactic reaction.

Anaphylaxis is a rare yet almost immediate and extreme allergic response. Common symptoms are dizziness, a sudden decrease in blood pressure, a swollen throat, heart palpitations, and a feeling that you are going to faint. If not treated immediately, anaphylaxis can be life-threatening.

Those who have a tendency toward anaphylaxis, whether in response to food sensitivity or insect bites, should always carry an EpiPen (epinephrine auto-injector) or an Insect Ana-Kit with them. These kits are used to inject a small dose of medication to stop the reaction. Check with your doctor, who can tell you when and how to use them.

There are no known cures for food allergies and intolerances. Avoidance is the best solution. This is easy enough to do at home, where you can prepare your own food, but it can sometimes prove difficult when eating in restaurants. Chefs often like to disguise various ingredients in their dishes, especially sauces and salads,

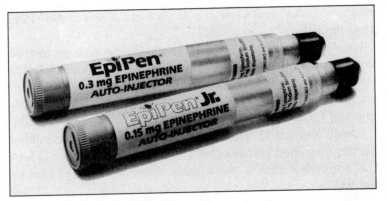

EpiPen. (*Center Laboratories*)

or they will mix together unusual food combinations. If you know that you're sensitive to a particular item, be sure to inquire how dishes are prepared and what ingredients went into them.

Always be vigilant! I was once having dinner in a French restaurant in New York with a friend who has an anaphylactic reaction to mushrooms. He inquired to make sure that none of the sauces had mushrooms and placed his order accordingly. Later, as we were eating, he discovered a sliver of mushroom mixed in with his peas. The kitchen apologized profusely, explaining that the chef often used the same spoon to dish out the various vegetables and by accident a piece of mushroom had landed in with the peas. Had my friend ingested that one innocent-looking little mushroom slice he could easily have become very sick.

Former Olympians John Powell and Doug Padilla both have asthma and are highly sensitive to many different foods. Both have also used a change of diet to help combat their asthma and bring about improvement in their athletic performances.

Powell, a burly, well-conditioned discus thrower, is renowned for both his superb throwing ability and his longevity in the sport. He was a member of four Olympic teams from 1972 through 1988, capturing bronze medals in 1976 and 1984. In 1975 he set a world record with a throw of 226 feet, 8 inches. Powell also posted the longest throws in the world in 1974, 1981, 1984, and 1987 and was the U.S. National Champion in 1974 and 1975 and again from 1983 through 1987.

Looking at John Powell you see power and strength, yet in 1985 Powell had a big asthma scare immediately after competing in a track meet in Eugene, Oregon, and thought he was going to die. "I couldn't breathe," he says. "It felt like someone had me in a vise grip and I was slowly being strangled."

Powell was quickly taken to a local hospital, where one of the doctors diagnosed him as asthmatic. Powell was surprised to hear this, for he had recently been under a doctor's care for allergies but had never suspected that he also had asthma.

From 1975 to 1983, Powell had been treated for allergies to ragweed, pollen, and various other substances and received seven allergy shots a week. Then, in 1983, he began seeing a physician near his home in San Jose, California. He was put through a battery of tests and found to be intolerant to forty-three different foods, including milk, wheat, soy, and eggs. Powell has since cut down on some of these foods and eliminated others from his diet. In their place, he's substituted a lot of fruits and vegetables and more than eight glasses of water a day.

Today, the forty-year-old Powell no longer takes allergy shots and is only minimally bothered by his allergies. "If I do start feeling some of the familiar symptoms like a runny nose, itchiness, or depression," says Powell, "I can usually nip it in the bud by owning up to the fact that I've been overdoing it with certain foods. So I'll quickly cut down or eliminate them and increase my water intake to flush out my system. This gives me a certain amount of control over my allergies."

Powell admits that there are times when he's strongly tempted to go off the diet. "It's tough always having to say no to things you like to eat. But then you've got a decision to make: What's more important—competing at your full potential or eating a particular food? I tell myself that I'd rather compete. And that's enough to make me stick to my diet."

In 1985, Doug Padilla, a runner, was rated number two in the world in the 5,000 meters. All that year he lost only one race—to Sidney Maree, an American runner whom he beat the next four times they met. After a spectacular 1985, Padilla was looking forward to an even better 1986. Instead, 1986 turned out to be a major disappointment for him. His best time that year for the 5,000 was a full thirty seconds slower than his best in 1985, and he quickly tumbled down through the rankings to number thirty.

Padilla couldn't account for this drastic change in his running. Something was sapping him of his strength, and he no longer possessed the reserves required for a fast race. Whenever the pace quickened, he was unable to keep up. "At the beginning of a race, I'd always start out tired. I felt as though I had already run a mile or two," Padilla recalls. "I had no gas. The other runners would begin to move and I'd try to move with them but I couldn't."

Padilla had had childhood asthma and bad allergies since he was two years old. "There were four of us in the family, all with allergies, but I was the only one with asthma." Padilla had received

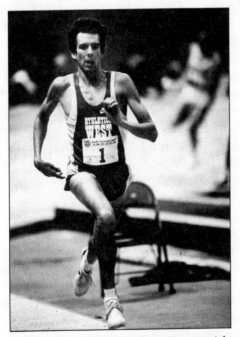

Doug Padilla. (R. M. Collins III, copyright © 1986)

allergy shots since he was seven, continuing with them for fourteen years. After his poor performances in 1986, it occurred to him that allergies or asthma might be at the root of his troubles. He consulted an allergist near his home in Orem, Utah, and was put on a medication program that included the asthma medications Intal, Ventolin, and Nasalcrom. The drugs cleared up his hay fever symptoms and the congestion in his chest, but the extreme fatigue that he had experienced prior to taking the medication persisted.

At the end of 1986, Padilla began seeing a physician in Aspen, Colorado, who discovered that Padilla was highly sensitive to numerous foods and food additives. He put the runner on a restrictive diet that dramatically changed his eating habits. Padilla stopped consuming simple carbohydrates and milk products and limited his intake of beef.

Since starting on this elimination diet, Padilla says that he feels much better. He did well at the U.S. Olympic trials in the summer of 1988 and made the Olympic team, getting as far as the semifinals at the Olympics in Seoul. Though not entirely satisfied with his showing in Seoul, he feels it represents a major improvement over his 1986 performances and most of those in 1987.

"Since switching to my new doctor, my workouts are moving more and more in the direction of 1985," Padilla says. "But it takes awhile to get everything back in balance. I know that I'll still have trouble with my allergies some days but at least it won't be as bad as it was before. With the diet, my body's apparently much better able to handle them."

Sulfites

The chemical additive sulfite can trigger asthma. It is listed on canned and bottled goods as potassium and sodium bisulfite, sulfur dioxide, sodium sulfite, or potassium or sodium metabisulfite. While sulfites have proved very useful as a preservative, they are also a common trigger for 5 to 10 percent of people with asthma. (See Appendix C.)

The use of sulfites as food preservatives is widespread, and products do not always have labels to identify them. Salad bars often use sulfites to prevent the discoloration of vegetables and to enhance color. If you're sensitive to sulfites, be sure to ask about them in restaurants before filling your plate. Sulfites are also put on many different fruits, vegetables, fish (especially shrimp), dried fruit, and in dips (especially those containing avocado), many commercially prepared baked goods, and even some nebulized (mist) asthma medications such as Bronkosol, Isuprel, and Metaprel. All wines contain sulfites, too. Check their labels carefully.

Typically, a short while after an allergic person eats something containing sulfites, a reaction sets in, resulting in hives, nausea, or diarrhea. Sulfites can bring on an asthma episode as well as induce anaphylaxis in some people.

Tartrazine

Another common food additive to be aware of if you have asthma is tartrazine, also known as Yellow Food Dye #5. This food coloring can be found in a wide range of products, including soft drinks, candies, cereals, baked goods, and some medications. Tartrazine can trigger an asthma episode and is particularly troublesome for people whose asthma is aggravated by aspirin.

As with sulfites, learn to become a label reader if you think you may be sensitive. Check what ingredients are in a product before you buy or eat it. If the ingredients aren't listed and you have your doubts, play it safe and choose another product.

ASPIRIN AND OTHER MEDICATIONS

Common aspirin is the most widely used medication in America. However, two in a thousand people have varying degrees of allergic reaction to it. It's believed that 8 to 20 percent of all people with asthma also have a hypersensitivity to aspirin. Within thirty minutes of taking aspirin or a product containing aspirin, aspirin-sensitive asthmatics (ASA) can develop runny noses, swollen eyes, or severe asthma.

If you have asthma and a sensitivity to aspirin, it's best to avoid the product completely, using suitable substitutes such as acetaminophen (Tylenol, Datril), which won't aggravate your asthma. Be sure to read the labels of all questionable products carefully for traces of aspirin. The more common products with aspirin include: Alka-Seltzer, Anacin, Bayer Aspirin, Bufferin, Ecotrin, Empirin, Excedrin, Midol, and Percodan.

Two other types of medication pose serious problems for people with asthma: beta-blockers and sedatives. Beta-blockers are frequently prescribed to decrease heart activity, control angina, and reduce high blood pressure. A possible side effect is constriction of the air passages. Among the most commonly prescribed beta-blockers are Inderal, Lopressor, Inderide, and Blocadren. If you take a beta-blocker, make sure that you bring this to the attention of both the cardiologist and the doctor who treats you for asthma.

People with asthma usually should not take sedatives, tranquilizers, or sleeping pills, even if they are experiencing only slight asthma symptoms. These drugs can lead not only to a worsening of the symptoms, but to death as well. The most commonly prescribed sedatives are Valium, Thorazine, and Librium. Sedatives and barbiturates used to relieve some of the anxiety that asthma can produce can instead dull and slow the respiratory system, making it even more difficult to breathe. As the breathing apparatus grows less and less efficient, the person with asthma can lose consciousness and die from lack of oxygen. Always check with your asthma doctor about sedatives if another physician prescribes them for you.

EMOTIONS

Asthma may be *triggered* by emotional responses such as anger, fear, laughter, or sadness, but, contrary to popular perception, it is *not caused* by emotional reactions. Asthma is physiological in nature, not psychosomatic, and the idea that asthma is "all in your head" is a wrong assumption that has haunted people with asthma for far too long. Just as you wouldn't tell a disabled person to get out of the wheelchair and walk across the room, you shouldn't tell a person with asthma to "just breathe."

People with asthma have hypersensitive airways and may develop some asthma following an extreme emotion such as laughter or sorrow. These emotions can lead to a change in breathing pattern that then can trigger bronchospasm.

IRRITANTS

Tobacco

Keith Brantley, the long-distance runner, claims that his lungs are so sensitive to tobacco smoke that when he goes for a run on a road and a car passes him, he can actually tell whether someone in the car is smoking a cigarette. When my swimming team practiced outdoors in a pool, if any spectator on the pool deck lit up a cigarette, almost on cue the entire team would stop swimming and begin looking around for the culprit. And I was one of the only ones on the team who had asthma!

Cigarette smoke is an especially acute problem for someone with asthma. Riding in airplanes and elevators without proper ventilation or dining in restaurants that don't offer separate nonsmoking areas can bring on distress. Secondary smoke from cigarettes, even just lingering traces of it, is enough to trigger an asthma episode by causing receptors in the nose and throat to constrict.

People with asthma can take steps to avoid tobacco smoke. Most of the time, with a little effort and vigilance, they will be successful. However, there are occasions when slightly more aggressive measures are called for. Dr. Manuel Sanguily, the Masters swimming champion and former Olympian, remembers a time when he encountered a special problem at work.

Two new workers in the office adjoining Sanguily's were chain-smokers who frequently indulged their habit in the corridor. Each time Sanguily stepped into the hall he would begin to cough and wheeze. After months of politely explaining what cigarette smoke could do to people with asthma, after numerous requests that his new neighbors at least restrict their tobacco habit to their own office without response, Sanguily decided to take action. One morning he quietly slipped a note under his neighbors' door. Within a few days he noticed that the volume of smoke in the halls had lessened considerably. Dr. Sanguily's message read as follows: "Thank you for not smoking. Cigarette smoke is the residue of your pleasure. It pollutes the air, contaminates my hair, and dirties my clothes, not to mention what it does to my lungs. This takes place without my consent. I have a pleasure also. I like a beer now and then. The residue of my pleasure is urine. Would you be annoyed if I stood on a chair and, without your consent, pissed on your head?"

TOBACCO AND THE EXERCISER

Although it's quite possible for smokers who have asthma to perform adequately at tennis, to compete in running races, and to participate in other sports, it goes without saying that they'd perform at much higher levels and be in considerably better health if they didn't use tobacco products. Athletes and sports groups recognize the importance of giving up tobacco. So should smokers with asthma, who by quitting would possibly require less medication and lead longer, healthier lives.

"Carbon monoxide and tars are the harmful substances in cigarettes," explains Tom Ferguson, M.D., a medical writer and former smoker from Austin, Texas. "People smoke for the nicotine, an addictive substance, but they die from the tars and carbon monoxide. Although nicotine tricks the body into relaxing by releasing substances in the brain, it's really only exercise that can truly relax the body's muscles naturally."

WHAT HAPPENS WHEN YOU SMOKE

The carbon monoxide in cigarettes retards athletic performance because it causes the hemoglobin molecule in the blood, a molecule that regularly carries oxygen to fuel the body's muscles and tissues, to pick up carbon monoxide molecules instead. It's estimated that by smoking one pack of cigarettes a day, you cut your blood's oxygen-carrying capacity by 10 percent. To make up for this oxygen deficit, your heart and lungs have to work overtime in order to produce the normal amount.

For the person with asthma, someone whose lungs already have to work overtime during certain periods, the body's oxygen supply diminishes. Smoking means even more work for the heart and lungs and ultimately less oxygen for your body. Also, smoking, unlike asthma, can permanently damage the lungs.

Just think how much healthier a person with asthma is when he or she doesn't smoke! And some of the results can be immediate. When a person quits smoking, carbon monoxide disappears from the body in about two to three days. Within a week that person is back down to the levels of a nonsmoker. The cancer-related risks associated with smoking will also go down to the baseline levels of nonsmokers, but that often takes years.

HELP IN QUITTING

The following groups offer help and information about how to stop smoking:

- *Smoker's Health Update* is a bulletin that includes summaries of the latest smoking research and descriptions of self-care approaches for smokers. The *Update* also contains reviews of products to help smokers quit. For more information, contact Smoker's Health Update, 3805 Stevenson Avenue, Austin, TX 78703.
- The American Lung Association has two guides for quitting smoking, *Freedom from Smoking in 20 Days*, and *A Lifetime of Freedom from Smoking*. Contact the association for information at 1740 Broadway, New York, NY 10019, 212-315-8700.
- Fresh Start is the name of the four-session program offered by local affiliates of the American Cancer Society to help people give up smoking. For information about joining, or to receive the free booklet, *I Quit Kit*, contact the local office of the American Cancer Society listed in your phone book.

Other Common Irritants

In addition to cigarette smoke, there are many other everyday household products and substances that can trigger an asthmatic episode. Among these are detergents, cosmetics, perfumes, paints, glues, ammonia, cleaning fluids, plaster dust, newsprint, and gasoline fumes. Although it's nearly impossible to avoid all of these items on a daily basis, it will help if you closely monitor your symptoms and keep a brief record, so that you and your doctor will have a better chance of isolating the main offenders. *The Asthma Organizer* is an excellent diary. Contact Mothers of Asthmatics, Inc. (10875 Main Street, Suite 210, Fairfax, VA 22030, 703-385-4403).

If you have asthma, often you will discover that your symptoms are more pronounced away from home—at school or work—or while engaging in a particular hobby. Try to determine what triggers may be present in these places by noting differences between your home and the other environment, and then take appropriate steps to avoid them.

WEATHER, CLIMATE, AIR POLLUTION

Asthma episodes can also be triggered by exposure to different types of air or by a sudden change in the air temperature or quality. Christine Dakin, of the Martha Graham Dance Company in New York City, describes her asthma as so sensitive to temperature variation that simply going indoors or outdoors will set off a fit of sneezing and coughing and bring on watery eyes.

Even air-conditioning can sometimes be hazardous. Keith Brantley, the runner, has found that competing indoors in Florida and other warm-weather sites around the country usually presents a problem for him because the extremely dry air produced by industrial-size air-conditioning systems makes his lungs close up. A particularly harrowing experience happened several years ago after Brantley finished a race in an air-conditioned arena in Florida. He was being interviewed by a reporter when he suddenly began coughing uncontrollably. Seconds later he was lying flat on his back on the ground and his condition came close to being life-threatening. Brantley believes that he didn't die that night because his lungs were so strong and well trained from all the aerobic work he put them through while running.

Many people with asthma are sensitive to more than one type of temperature change or weather condition. Finding the right time and place to train can pose problems that athletes without asthma just don't have to contend with. Shirley Dery-Batlik, a member of the 1984 U.S. Olympic canoeing and kayaking team, used to be bothered by hot, humid air as well as very cold air. For the last few years, however, only cold weather has given her trouble. Her worst symptom is an especially hard and deep cough, which can even cause her to vomit. "By the way that I cough you'd think I was a smoker," she says. Once, after a particularly harrowing coughing incident, she popped a blood vessel in her eye.

In order to get through her workouts with a minimum of hacking and inconvenience, Dery-Batlik wears a cotton bandana over her nose and mouth (cops-and-robbers style) whenever the weather is bad. This gives her nose a chance to warm the frigid air before it hits her lungs.

Cold Air

Inhaling cold air that is not first warmed and humidified by the nasal passages causes the bronchial tubes to constrict. This happens in a mild form to everyone. If a person with asthma continues to breathe frigid air, however, the bronchospasms may intensify. Exercising in the cold will often bring on a swifter asthma episode, because during exercise, breaths are generally deeper and more rapid than during sedentary activities.

HOW TO EXERCISE IN COLD WEATHER

If you're affected by cold-air-induced bronchospasm, it's best to:

- Premedicate before you are exposed to cold, dry air.

- Set aside extra time for a longer warm-up to prepare your lungs properly.
- Try to breathe through your nose as much as possible instead of through your mouth. Your nose is much better at warming and humidifying the cold air.
- Cover your mouth and nose with either a scarf or a ski mask to warm the air as it enters the body.
- On days when the thermometer plummets, consider an alternative indoor workout.

Dry Air

While northern winters are intolerable for many people with asthma, the warm, exceedingly dry areas of the country are just as troublesome for others. In dry areas, humidifiers are highly recommended to keep air moist and the air passages well hydrated. Be sure to clean humidifiers on a regular basis to prevent mold and bacterial growth, both of which can trigger asthma in some people. Caution must also be used with ultrasonic humidifiers because they may disperse minerals into the air, which can then be inhaled and cause irritation.

Humid, Hot Air

The water suspended in humid air carries all kinds of possible allergens with it. While the moist air may be beneficial for the lungs, it provides an excellent avenue for dust, pollens, and molds to find their way into your airways. If you're bothered by this type of weather, try to avoid it by staying indoors as much as possible on hot, humid days. Use your clean air conditioner and/or an electrostatic air filter indoors.

A study of children carried out at a research center in Israel found that asthma episodes flared up greatly from midday to late afternoon. Researchers discovered that temperature and humidity rose by as much as one-third from morning to late afternoon, and that this was the time when children were most active and outdoors the most.

If either you or your child is affected by changes in temperature and humidity, it's recommended that you not exercise outdoors between midday and late afternoon or that you medicate at midday before exercising outdoors.

Other Weather Conditions

Some people find that their asthma flares up when the temperature and barometric pressure change rapidly. Others have more problems on windy days, when pollen is more likely to be airborne. Some find relief on rainy days because the rain tends to cleanse the air, improving its quality.

Obviously, a wide range of weather conditions will affect different people, depending on each individual's triggers. The best remedy: Know yourself and be prepared for possible reactions by listening to weather forecasts.

Keep a daily diary and make special note not only of your sensitivities but also of the specific weather conditions on that particular day. In addition to troublesome days, note down days that you remain symptom-free. By being able to pinpoint fairly accurately what type of weather bothers you the most, you'll be able to take measures to avoid an asthma flare-up.

Air Pollution

Bonnie Warner, a member of the U.S. luge team in the 1984 and 1988 Winter Olympics, still occasionally has asthma episodes when the weather is cold. "But that's nothing compared to all the problems I had with asthma as a child," admits Warner.

Warner attended junior high school in Upland, California, which is located in a valley that is continually filled with smog. "For three straight years in the mid-seventies, Upland was rated the smoggiest town in the Western Hemisphere because of all the air pollution that blew in from Los Angeles," recalls Warner. "When

I started junior high there, I went out for the cross-country team, but that proved to be a really big mistake! I wasn't able to adjust to the bad air, which is something no one should have to do anyway, and I got sick. Because of the polluted air, I ended up missing half the school year with asthma."

Today Warner has mostly outgrown her asthma, but there are times when heavy air pollution can still trigger it, and then she usually exercises indoors, as do countless other asthmatic athletes, because of the increasing air-pollution levels nationwide.

Unfortunately, for those who are bothered by poor air quality in their hometown, moving to a place free of man-made pollutants such as smog and emissions from smokestacks and industrial plants may be the only solution to the problem.

Athletes traveling to compete in areas with low levels of air quality should also take extra precautions:

- Check with your physician to see if you need an increase in medication dosage or change in medication.
- Spend extra time warming up in an air-conditioned area prior to competition.
- Train and/or compete while wearing a mask.

OZONE POLLUTION AND EXERCISE

Outdoor exercisers around the country have not had particularly good summers these past few years due to the elevated air-pollution levels. Some people have found it physically painful to work out at times, causing many of them to check the ozone levels in their regions before deciding whether it makes sense to exercise. And these are people without asthma!

Ozone, once thought to be a health problem only for southern California, now constitutes a large portion of summertime air pollution for the New York City metropolitan area, Denver, Chicago, Detroit, and many other large cities. If ozone levels continue to increase, the outlook for summertime exercise will be grim not only for people with asthma but for everyone.

Ozone is an invisible vapor produced in the lower atmosphere through a complex chemical reaction of sunlight, hydrocarbons from automobile exhaust, and nitrogen oxides, which also come from auto exhaust and from power-plant emissions. Only a change in the weather, more wind, rain, or cooler temperatures, for example, will clear this unhealthful air from the region.

"Ozone may be approaching cigarette smoking as a factor affecting health," says Morton Lippmann, Ph.D., professor of environmental medicine at the New York University Medical Center in Manhattan. "While there certainly may be benefits from exercising, if you exercise in ozone you're counteracting those benefits."

According to Lippmann, if you don't have asthma and regularly exercise when ozone levels are high, you may experience chest tightness, find it difficult to breathe, or have headaches. Your workout level may also drop. For someone with asthma, wheezing or more serious complications may be triggered by ozone inhalation. But the real health problems for everyone, says Dr. Lippmann, might appear later when young exercisers turn fifty or sixty years old and then discover they have breathing difficulties similar to emphysema.

The federal Environmental Protection Agency has set an ozone standard of 0.12 parts per million as a safety border. In theory, when ozone levels are tested daily and found to be below this level, you can safely exercise outdoors. However, when it's hot and sunny and levels rise above this limit, you'd certainly be a lot safer staying indoors watching TV with the air conditioner on.

Some criticize the federal ozone safety standard for not being protective enough. "Healthy children and adults who exercise can experience health-related effects from ozone even at or below these federal levels," says Judy Schreiber, a research scientist with the New York State Health Department in Albany. "There's really no margin of safety in the level."

Some people experience trouble with ozone when the level is well below the federal standard because sensitivity to ozone varies enormously from person to person. Unfortunately, to date there's no real way to predict who can tolerate ozone, who can't, and at what levels ozone poses a health risk for most people.

While an exerciser can readily learn to tolerate and adapt to extreme heat as well as to high altitudes with no long-term health consequences, it's certainly not advisable to go out for a run or a training ride on your bike in an attempt to get used to ozone pollution. "Continuing to exercise and adapt to ozone will get you past the initial symptoms of ozone and your reduced athletic performance," says Dr. Lippmann, "but this adaptation won't protect you from the cumulative, long-term damage from the pollution. When you inhale ozone deeper into your lungs, it destroys cells, and the effects are irreversible."

What are your exercise options in this new ozone-pollution era that seems to be dawning on many American cities? As ozone pollution continues to rise to unhealthful levels, it's becoming more useful to consult the Pollution Standard Index (PSI) before heading out for a workout. "When the ozone levels are high you should really exercise outdoors before ten A.M., before the ozone has a chance to build up," says Dr. Lippmann. "Once ozone-pollution levels are elevated, they generally stay high until early evening."

Other exercise options include moving your workouts indoors, working out late at night, or simply cutting back exercise activities whenever pollution levels are elevated. Also, since ozone pollution is relatively low in the fall, winter, and early spring, it's better to perform your more strenuous workouts at these times of year instead of in the summertime.

There is no health benefit to exercising outdoors when air-pollution levels are high. When in doubt about the current air quality, contact the regional office of your state Department of Environmental Conservation. Ask for the current PSI level. This numerical reading, which is generally checked several times during the day, takes into account the ozone level for the region as well as other air-pollution factors. It can serve as a good indicator of whether it's safe enough for strenuous exercise.

Pollution Standard Index (PSI)

0–50	=	GOOD*
50–99	=	MODERATE*
100–199	=	UNHEALTHFUL
200–299	=	VERY UNHEALTHFUL
300–500	=	HAZARDOUS

*It's safe to exercise

SOURCE: New York State Environmental Conservation Department

OZONE ALERT

The following metropolitan areas exceeded the federal standard for ozone pollution in 1987. Also included here are the number of days the standard was exceeded:

Los Angeles 48	Atlanta 15
Bakersfield, Calif. 48	Sacramento 15
Fresno, Calif. 43	Chicago 13
San Diego 27	Milwaukee 13
Philadelphia 23	Connecticut River Valley 12
Visalia, Calif. 22	Baltimore 11
Houston 21	El Paso 11
Modesto, Calif. 21	Muskegon, Mich. 11
New York City 19	Washington, D.C. 11

SOURCE: Environmental Protection Agency

COLDS AND OTHER
RESPIRATORY INFECTIONS

If I were to look at my body as a machine, my lungs would be the weak link, the part that is undependable and needs the most attention and pampering. It's the same with so many other people like me who have asthma. We happen to be a good deal more susceptible to colds and other types of respiratory infections than average people. Just why this is so is not precisely understood by doctors, but recent research indicates that the answer may have much to do with the large buildup of mucus in the airways, where infections can more easily take hold. For some, especially children, asthma will be triggered within days (sometimes just hours) of coming down with a cold or flu. Very often asthma symptoms will linger even after the infection has cleared up.

Christine Dakin, the Martha Graham troupe member, finds that her asthma is almost always triggered by flulike symptoms and a run-down feeling. For this reason, she is wary of the other dancers in the company when they begin sneezing or coughing or complaining of a scratchy throat, and she then does her best to avoid them temporarily, though it's often difficult to manage. She understands herself well enough to know that once she comes down with a bug it could mean weeks and weeks of trouble with her asthma, valuable time missed at rehearsals, and possibly a trip to the hospital.

Dakin, now thirty-seven, first developed asthma at the age of twenty-six. Although she was asthma-free as a child, she recalls that she frequently had bronchitis and believes that this may well have been a forerunner of her asthma. Much like myself, Christine may also have had undiagnosed asthma.

There are times when a bad upper respiratory infection, either viral or bacterial, will suddenly trigger asthma in someone who never had it before. Dr. Jim Angel, chairman of the Department of Health and Physical Education at Samford University in Birmingham, Alabama, was at sea serving his commission in the navy (after graduating from the Naval Academy at Annapolis two and a half

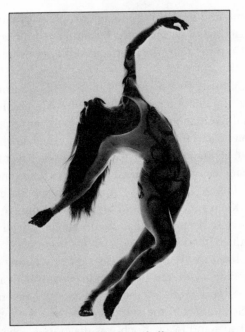

Christine Dakin. (*Chuck Kimball*)

years earlier) when, without warning, he had his first asthma episode. Angel cannot say with absolute certainty what triggered the asthma, but his strong guess is that it was the bad chest cold he had developed while on the ocean.

"I was working ten-to-sixteen-hour days on the ship and my resistance was down," Angel says. "I started wheezing and feeling this strange shortness of breath. I had no idea what it was except that it wasn't normal. As soon as we docked in Naples, Italy, I was sent to the naval hospital. They diagnosed my asthma and a short time later I was medically discharged from the navy."

It's unfortunate that Angel's career, like countless other military careers, was cut short by a stringent policy that excludes anyone who has asthma. The U.S. Military Academy and the U.S. Naval Academy exclude any candidates who have had any asthma past the age of thirteen. In this era of better asthma diagnosis, medical management, and medical follow-up, people with asthma are still being discriminated against based on antiquated conceptions about asthma. It's time that the military policy was reviewed and changed.

Bill Koch, thirty-two, winner of the 1982 Cross Country World Cup skiing title and a member of the 1984 Winter Olympic team, also traces the initial onset of his asthma to upper respiratory problems. When he was fifteen years old, Koch came down with a very serious case of strep throat, a bacterial infection. Over the next two to three years, he had strep throat three more times and bronchitis ten times. In the winter of 1974, these infections evolved into asthma, as Koch suddenly found himself struggling to finish races at nowhere near his potential and with his lungs feeling as if they were "completely on fire."

Koch realized that something was seriously wrong and hurried from his home in Vermont to Boston to consult with a pulmonary specialist. After a thorough medical exam and several treadmill tests, which duplicated the symptoms he had been experiencing in his workouts and races, Koch was diagnosed as having asthma and given medication to help him manage it.

Sinus infections can also make asthma worse, and if they are not brought to the attention of your doctor and properly treated, they may keep triggering asthma flare-ups on a regular basis. Long-distance-running star Keith Brantley has found that his system builds up mucus twice as heavily whenever he has a cold. As a result, even after the cold has cleared up, his sinuses continue to bother him for weeks. This affects his training and makes it that much harder and takes that much longer for him to work himself back into peak condition.

George Murray, the top wheelchair athlete from Florida, had chronic sinusitis for many years, which in turn complicated his asthma. At first, Murray's doctors treated him with antibiotics, but after a point these proved ineffective. They then tried irrigating his sinuses by inserting tiny rubber hoses into his forehead. This didn't work either, and as a last-ditch effort, the infected sinuses were removed surgically, which did provide him with relief.

Pushing Yourself

Many athletes and coaches follow the "No pain, no gain" philosophy for workouts. Disregarding body signals that tell them that they're injured or seriously fatigued, athletes push themselves or are urged by their coaches through a workout or competition, often becoming more fatigued and needing extra time to recover, or else aggravating their injury to such an extent that it sets back their recovery time considerably. Obviously, this is not the kind of pain that brings about any gain.

It's important for exercisers or athletes to realize that there are two types of "pain" that they may confront in a workout. How well they are able to distinguish the two types can often have an overriding effect on their entire season. One kind of pain involves muscle fatigue and the "burn" they feel in their muscles during a particularly hard workout or competition. This burn is actually caused during the anaerobic phase, in which the working muscle tissue is flooded with lactic acid, a waste material, which then causes a "burning" sensation in the tissue. The other pain active exercisers can feel comes if they try to push their body through a workout when they're injured or have an illness or fever.

I've found that there is no limit to the first kind of pain, and being able to train your muscles to work as efficiently as possible even though they are fatigued is a way to build endurance and make progress as an athlete. On the other hand, I stop swim workouts immediately whenever I feel the first twinge of pain in my shoulder or feel that I've reached a point where my asthma is coming on. In times of pain like this, it doesn't help you become a better athlete if you continue to push your body through a workout. Whatever is bothering you will only get worse if you continue to exercise, and could set your training back for an indefinite period.

It pays always to be aware of your asthma status. If you feel your asthma is particularly aggravated by colds and flus, then ease up a bit on your exercise program if you have the sniffles, body aches, or feel particularly run-down. You might even consider eliminating a workout or two until you feel completely better. There is nothing wimpish about this. A world-class athlete pushes his or her body in one sense, but knows how to baby it as well. Remember, it's better to miss a couple of workouts and take care of your asthma than to miss a few weeks or possibly even your entire season because you tried to "play through" it.

Colds: A Note on Medication

You've heard it before: We can put a man on the moon, but we can't cure the common cold. To date, there is no medicine that can prevent colds. However, there are flu vaccinations that are often successful in preventing the current season's popular type of flu if taken prior to the "flu season."

Bronchitis and bacterial infections such as pneumonia and strep throat go hand in hand with asthma for many people, especially me. When a person with asthma who has a history of dual conditions (asthma triggered by colds, viruses, or bronchitis) develops any of these infections, his or her asthma physician should be alerted in order to begin mounting a counteroffensive.

Your doctor will take a detailed history, listen to your chest, and take a culture test if strep throat is suspected. If you do indeed have a bacterial infection, antibiotics will be prescribed for a ten-day period to kill the bacteria. Even if you're feeling great after the first few days, be sure to finish the antibiotics. The bacteria may only be weakened at first, and if you stop taking the medication, it may rebound in your system and pose even more serious health problems.

Remember that colds and flus are viral infections. Medicating yourself with antibiotics (which are only effective in treating *bacterial* infections) will do nothing to eliminate a cold or flu. Also, if you have asthma and are sensitive to antibiotics, you might induce a reaction and have an asthma episode. Therefore, always check with your physician before medicating yourself.

7

EXERCISE-INDUCED BRONCHOSPASM

$\mathbf{E}$xercise is the most common of all the known asthma triggers after allergies, affecting an estimated 60 percent to 90 percent of people who have asthma. If an asthmatic performs an athletic movement—this could be running, skiing, swimming, cycling, basketball, or aerobic dance—for at least five minutes at 70 percent of his or her aerobic capacity, he or she can trigger exercise-induced bronchospasm (EIB), or exercise-induced asthma (EIA), as it's also called.

EIB, if untreated, can severely hamper athletic performance. It's also enough to keep many people from exercising out of fear that they will trigger an asthma episode. There's no reason for this; everyone can be aerobically fit if they want to be. Current research suggests that those with asthma who have improved their aerobic fitness are better able to cope with airway obstruction than untrained persons with the same degree of obstruction or severity of asthma. And that's good news for asthmatics who want a good reason to be in shape.

If you have EIB but are sitting on the sidelines, just remember that EIB is reversible through proper management. If you do want to exercise, EIB no longer has to be an excuse to keep you from starting or continuing with an exercise or sports program.

WHAT CAUSES EIB?

Asthma researchers know what happens once EIB occurs, but after years of study they are still uncertain as to why it happens in the first place.

Francois Haas, director of the Pulmonary Function Laboratory at New York University School of Medicine, offers this explanation: "As a person begins to take in air more and more rapidly to meet the demands of the sport or exercise he's engaged in, the air is less likely to be properly warmed and humidified as it passes through the nose and mouth and into the lungs. The effect of this colder, drier air on the airways is believed to actually trigger an asthma flare."

SYMPTOMS

EIB can occur in people like me who are rarely bothered by asthma except when they exercise. But it can also occur in people whose asthma is triggered by other factors such as allergies. It affects both children and adults who try to be active. Symptoms can range from mild to extreme depending on the individual, the type of exercise, and presence of other triggers, which seem to abound when you exercise outdoors during pollen season. They become noticeable within five minutes after exercise is begun and reach their peak five to ten minutes after exercise has stopped. Depending on the severity of the reaction, recovery is usually complete in thirty to ninety minutes. Hospitalization is rarely necessary with EIB. However, repeated bouts may make the lungs more reactive to another trigger.

EIB symptoms include shortness of breath, coughing, wheezing, a "tight" or "burning" feeling in the chest, abdominal pain, headaches, and fatigue. If the individual had normal lung function before starting to exercise, the symptoms will generally clear up by

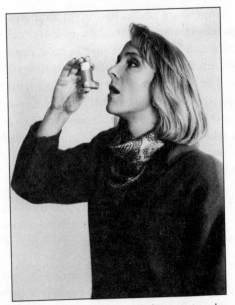

Many exercisers use an inhaler twenty minutes before they begin their workout.

themselves. If not, the use of an inhaled bronchodilator to expand the airways will generally stop an episode within minutes. However, I recommend that if you are going to exercise, you use your medicine prophylactically: Take your prescribed puffs twenty to thirty minutes *prior* to exercise or your oral medicine an hour prior to exercise.

ENVIRONMENTAL FACTORS AFFECTING EIB

Cold, Dry Air

For many exercisers, working out in a warm and humid environment is less likely to bring on EIB than exercising in a cold, dry climate. I suspect that's one of the reasons I wasn't diagnosed for so long: I was swimming and always breathing the perfect air just above the surface of the water.

When the temperature begins to drop in autumn and early winter, many exercisers start to complain of EIB. Francois Haas, as well as other researchers, believe that as cold, dry air is inhaled, it helps speed up moisture loss from the airways and brings on EIB episodes. For some EIB-prone athletes, all it takes is a slight drop in temperature—perhaps just the difference between going from the hot outdoors to an air-conditioned room or car—to trigger asthma. Any cooling effect on what are already hyperreactive, or "twitchy," airways can usually cause a problem.

In order to prevent EIB episodes, breathing through the nose (as opposed to breathing through the mouth) is recommended by athletes and asthma researchers. If the air is first taken in through the nose, it can be filtered, warmed, and moistened before it begins its journey to the pharynx, larynx, trachea, and finally to the bronchial tubes.

In the presence of cold air the mucous membranes of the nose automatically swell slightly to slow the passage of the air, allowing it to be humidified and then warmed. If, however, you begin to breathe in air directly through the mouth, you effectively bypass the filtering action of the nose and increase your susceptibility to EIB.

Many athletes who are adversely affected by cold air wear cold-weather masks, dust masks, or scarves around their nose and mouth when they go outside to train in cold weather. This extra protection keeps the inhaled air fairly warm and moist, and bronchospasm is minimized.

DIAGNOSING EIB

Many athletes are unaware, as I was for so many years, that they have EIB, and they continue to compete despite chest tightness, constant coughing, and wheezing. Others choose to "play through" their symptoms and not complain. Joan Pennington, a swimmer and member of the 1980 Olympic team for the 200-meter backstroke, is in this "denial" category. Often after a hard swim workout with the national team, her shoulders would turn purple from the strain of trying to take in air. When she runs six-minute miles, in training for the triathlons she now competes in, she sounds like someone on her last legs. "People stare at me because I make so much noise when I'm exercising," says Pennington. "I try hard to hide my breathing because it's so embarrassing, but it's not easy."

Although she found the constant wheezing irritating, Pennington refused to see a doctor about her asthma because she simply didn't like doctors. "I know it's an awful attitude," she admits, "but I only see them when I'm in bed, have a high fever, or I can't move." After talking with Joan at some length about this book, she was persuaded to see her doctor and now uses albuterol. "Now I think about running instead of breathing, and my legs get tired, not my lungs."

It's unfortunate that Joan, and countless other high-performance athletes like her, have this attitude about doctors and medication. I'm proof of what a good management program can do for one's performance and health, and I'm always reminding athletes with untreated asthma how much better they would feel if they finally took control of it, instead of being victimized by it.

Telltale EIB signals that can be picked up by an alert parent or coach include coughing during and after a workout, an initial good performance followed by a rapid drop-off (as EIB becomes apparent), and stomach cramps.

It has been demonstrated many times that athletic performance can increase dramatically if someone with undetected EIB is properly diagnosed and treated. This is especially important for children. "Many undiagnosed kids with EIB end up withdrawing completely from sports," says William E. Pierson, M.D., director of the Northwest Asthma and Allergy Center in Seattle, and an expert in EIB. "And those who don't withdraw will try their best to divert the active play of the entire athletic group to a more sedentary activity that they can then take part in."

Because sports can be such a socializing experience for children and teens, the family, along with the extended sports family—the coach, athletic trainer, sports physician, teammates, and athletic administration—should work together to make sure that all young people have the opportunity to learn and compete. It's on the playing fields that children learn about teamwork, goal setting, and how to postpone short-term gratification for long-term rewards.

TESTING FOR EIB

If EIB is suspected in a child or an adult, a board-certified allergist (a physician who has passed a special test administered by the American Board of Allergy and Immunology) or a pulmonologist can effectively test for it by having the patient run outside, ride a stationary bike, or use a treadmill or rowing machine for approximately five to eight minutes. During the office test, the physician will stand by with medication in case of emergency.

By using a stethoscope to listen to the patient's chest for wheezing and by taking a standard lung-function test (see chapter 8), a doctor will be able to determine if exercise is precipitating bronchospasm, and whether it's occurring in the large or smaller airways.

Who Should Be Screened for EIB?

While it's fairly accurate to say that 5 percent to 10 percent of all high-performance athletes will have bronchial hyperresponsiveness (an overreaction of the airways to some trigger), it would be a very costly procedure to screen every high-school, college, and professional athlete for EIB with a lab treadmill test. Many schools are now using a questionnaire in an effort to pick up probable asthma-risk athletes.

Certain factors can indicate that you may be predisposed to EIB. If you (or your child) are allergic, have hay fever, or have had asthma in the past, the chances are one in three that you have EIB as well, and you should be tested for its presence. You should also consider testing if you cough during or after exercise or seem unusually susceptible to bronchitis and colds.

PREVENTION AND CONTROL OF EIB: THE NONPHARMACOLOGICAL APPROACH

EIB shouldn't keep an athlete or exerciser on the sidelines. EIB can be controlled and prevented in most exercisers if steps are taken *before* a workout or competition begins. Nonpharmacological methods (those without medication) include the use of an extended warm-up session, special breathing techniques that can help minimize hyperventilation and promote relaxation, nasal breathing, wearing a mask, hypnotism, and keeping exercise to under an hour.

Many people with EIB don't have the option of using the nonpharmacological approach exclusively. What is outlined below may or may not work for you. Using as much of this approach as you can still has merits, however. Although I take medication, I also follow the steps in the nonpharmacological approach. Even if you know that you will be using medication, read this section for tips that you can use in addition to your medication program.

Use a Warm-up Period to Help Prevent EIB

In many cases, EIB symptoms start to develop five minutes after peak exercise exertion has started. Knowing this, many athletes in training choose to "run through" their wheezing, hacking, and coughing by starting out slowly and continuing to exercise at low intensity as the EIB comes on and finally subsides. Then they go into what's called a "refractory period"—a time when the stimulus of exercise won't trigger asthma so readily—and they're generally free to continue their workouts at high levels.

Other athletes start exercise at an intensity known to bring on EIB, step off to the sidelines to cough and/or wheeze, and then resume playing.

Many top athletes resist using medication because they dislike the side effects. "Some athletes often don't want other people to know that they have asthma," says Dr. Roger M. Katz, a clinical professor of pediatrics at the University of California at Los Angeles. Dr. Katz is also a board-certified allergist and treats many world-class athletes with asthma who train on the West Coast. He has found that many of the athletes he treats are embarrassed and don't want to take pills or be seen using an inhaler.

Some athletes think that asthma is a weakness—one that they'd rather not treat by taking medicine. They need to accept that asthma is not a weakness and that their athletic performance will be enhanced if they deal with the asthma and get it under control, rather than ignore it.

As outlined by Dr. Katz, a basic nonpharmacological approach for prevention of EIB consists of three distinct phases: pre-exercise, exercise, and post-exercise. Within the broad outline of the plan, an athlete and his or her physician have leeway to modify and personalize as they see fit. "Each athlete has his own endurance for how much exercise will cause the asthma," says Dr. Katz. "The patient has to realize this and try to find out what his tolerance level is."

For some people, the nonpharmacological approach works very nicely, says Dr. Katz. For others, it just doesn't have any effect. If the athlete who abhors medication tries the nonpharmacological approach and it doesn't work, this may pose problems. "Sometimes it may take an athlete quite a while to work through the feelings he has against taking medication to realize that it's okay to take some medication," says Dr. Katz. "One of the big problems that I have with elite athletes is that instead of taking asthma medication that I recommend, the athlete ends up taking something recommended by a peer or his coach. Unfortunately, the coaches, friends, and trainers are often misinformed."

Dr. Katz believes that by getting to the coaches and trainers first and educating them about asthma, a doctor can make great strides in developing a sense of trust with his patient/athlete. Only then will real progress be made.

Nonpharmacological Approach in
Preventing and Treating Exercise-Induced Bronchospasm

Pre-exercise	Exercise	Post-exercise
• 2 to 3 minutes of warm-up exercises followed by rest period • Warm-up can be as long as 40 minutes • Hypnosis	• Breathe warm, humid air • Breathe through your nose • Less than 5 minutes of maximum exertion	• Deep, slow breaths • 7 percent carbon dioxide inhalation, or rebreathe expired air in a paper bag • Repeat 5 minutes of exercise every 40 minutes

Pre-exercise

In the pre-exercise phase, you should begin warming up slowly to loosen the muscles and elevate the heart rate gradually. Once you begin to sweat lightly, you can perform your exercise activity at or close to your maximum exertion for up to five minutes and then take a rest.

Top athletes can continue with this warm-up for up to forty minutes and it's often enough to minimize the onset of EIB. Eventually, they are ready to go all out in their sport or exercise for an extended period.

Another warm-up routine consists of doing brief bouts of exercise or activity for two to three minutes followed by three minutes of rest. Again, for some people this may help prevent EIB symptoms by getting the lungs ready for exercise. "A good warm-up will often bring a smaller and smaller amount of bronchospasm until you get a refractory period," says Dr. Katz.

Before my own condition was diagnosed as asthma, I too discovered that if I warmed up longer at a higher intensity than my teammates, I'd swim faster in competition. My warm-ups sometimes lasted an hour. Also, if I swam several events in one day, I generally improved my performance as the day wore on. I also found that I needed an extra-long cool-down period. I would swim slowly until I had completely recovered, meaning I was relaxed and felt as if I hadn't competed at all that day.

These are general warm-up exercise outlines. You'll need to be flexible about your individual warm-up and know your own body and your personal threshold for exercising with asthma. You'll also have to adjust the amount of rest it takes for your bronchospasm to subside to fit your needs.

Dr. Katz has also found that hypnosis can help some athletes with asthma. While he's not an advocate of hypnotism, he's discovered that it can keep athletes from hyperventilating by relaxing them and can teach them to breathe more deeply and slowly by using their diaphragm.

Exercise Phase

Once an athlete has warmed up sufficiently and is in a refractory phase, the bulk of the workout can then begin. EIB symptoms can be reduced at this time by breathing warm, humid air rather than cold, dry air. If you are a swimmer, this generally isn't a problem if the pool temperature is in the 24-degree C or 80-degree F range. If you're riding a bike or out running, wearing a scarf or a cold weather mask (3M, available at most pharmacies) over your nose and mouth may help to humidify and warm the air that you take in.

Other athletes, says Dr. Katz, have learned to reduce EIB symptoms by breathing through their nose instead of their mouth. Admittedly, this is a hard technique to master for many, especially when you're at maximum exertion and literally start gulping for air.

Hyperventilation, breathing at an abnormally rapid rate, is thought to increase carbon dioxide loss, which then triggers EIB. "Many athletes get around hyperventilation by learning to breathe much deeper and more slowly," says Dr. Katz. "In many cases it seems to counter the effects of bronchospasm associated with hyperventilation." Mike Gminski, the center for the Philadelphia 76ers basketball team, regularly uses yogalike "belly breathing" to calm himself and bring a steady pattern to his breathing. (See chapter 10.)

The type of sport you play as well as your position can have an impact on your EIB susceptibility too. Sustained activities such as cross-country skiing, basketball, and long-distance running will often have a more negative impact on EIB symptoms than will swimming, bowling, football, weight lifting, and other typical stop-and-go activities.

Going all out in your sport or exercise routine in short bursts, each burst for less than five minutes at a stretch and with no more than forty minutes between them, seems to reduce the development of EIB as well.

Post-exercise

In the cool-down phase after your workout or competition, it's important to concentrate on breathing, making sure that you take deep, slow breaths. "Since carbon dioxide loss has been associated with bronchospasm," says Dr. Katz, "it's been found to be helpful for a small number of people to breathe back and forth into a paper bag, to stop their hyperventilating. This will either block or else change their asthma."

If you decide to go the nonpharmacological route, make sure you understand that there may come a point when you will have to accept medication in order to prevent serious asthma and associated illness. Not everyone, it must be pointed out, has side effects from medication. For those who do, however, and are bothered by them, the decision to forgo medication is one of the most important that they will have to make.

For two years the nonpharmacological approach seemed to work perfectly for cross-country skier Bill Koch, America's top racer, who won a silver medal at the 1976 Olympics in Innsbruck, Austria, in the 30-kilometer race. In 1982, Koch enhanced his reputation in the cross-country ski world by becoming the first American skier ever to win the World Cup, a difficult competition involving ten races that is held each winter on different courses around the world.

Koch's drug-free approach to EIB had been effective for him until two weeks before the start of the 1984 Winter Olympics in Sarajevo, Yugoslavia. It was then, due to a mistake on his part, that his asthma treatment plan backfired and ended up costing him an excellent opportunity for another Olympic medal.

Koch's asthma was first diagnosed in 1975 when he was nineteen years old. Koch's doctor started him on a medication program that consisted of cromolyn sodium, theophylline, and terbutaline, a beta-agonist. Although Koch was to take medication regularly for years, he never quite felt comfortable with it. "The side effects were bothersome and unpredictable from the very beginning," says Koch. "The medication raised my pulse and gave me an overall jittery feeling, especially when I took the pills.

"I took the medication every day for over six years, but there came a point when I was just no longer content with a drug solution to asthma and I began to look around for an alternative."

One autumn day in 1981, Koch simply quit taking his medication. "I was very pleased with myself for stopping," recalls Koch. "I made up my mind that day to really tune into my body and figure out how to manage the resources that were already there. I was determined to control my asthma without medication, and once I shifted my focus inward and learned to listen to my body, things became easy."

After careful analysis, Koch discovered exactly what triggered his asthma. The first trigger was exercising at high altitude, where the air wasn't nearly as humid as it was at sea level. The second trigger was a drop in the temperature to around 0 degrees. A third factor was having to compete on hilly courses.

The method Koch chose for dealing with altitude, frigid air, and hilly courses was to take an extra-long time in his warm-up, making sure that he raised his physical exertion level gradually whenever he had to practice or had a competition. Without the medication, it now became critical for him to develop, fine-tune, and then stick to a warm-up routine that would not only take his asthma into account, but also enable him to train and perform at peak potential.

If he didn't warm up properly, Koch found that he had only two choices. "I could either warm up during the race," he says, "but this meant starting slow and losing a lot of time. Or I could begin normally and eventually blow myself out because the pace was too fast for my asthma."

These were not viable options for a ski champion. "Once my asthma goes over the edge, it's virtually impossible to put things back together again for quite a while," says Koch. "By pushing my lungs too far, I can do some real damage, and then it often takes months for them to heal. Add in the cold-air factor and you can begin to see why the way I warmed up was so important."

To warm up, Koch would find a nice long hill and start to "ladder" himself up, going slowly from side to side with his skis, and then go back down again. Each time he did this, he took his pulse rate up a little higher, making sure that he never let it reach the point where he began to have difficulty breathing. "The whole time I was really listening closely to my body," says Koch.

With a lot of hard work, patience, and determination, Koch eventually thought he had perfected his warm-up routine and was little troubled by EIB after that. He had accomplished this while keeping his promise to himself to stay away from asthma medication, and in 1982 and 1983 he enjoyed the two best years of his career. Ironically, it was this success with his warm-up routine that led to his eventual troubles in 1984.

"I think I just became too complacent and overconfident," Koch admits upon reflection. "I started to feel that I had my asthma licked and that perhaps I had finally outgrown it. Since I wasn't getting the pain in my lungs anymore, I wasn't as vigilant and tuned in to the workings of my body as I should have been. In the end it really hurt me."

Two weeks before the 1984 Olympics, Koch "burned" his lungs very badly while competing in a race in Switzerland over a hilly, frigid, windblown setting, just the type of course and weather conditions that posed problems for his asthma. In addition, Koch had been quite ill the month before (not asthma related) and had lost important training time. As a result, he was nervous and overeager before the race.

"I blew it right there," Koch says. "I should never have raced in Switzerland after being so sick. It was really a gross case of mismanagement, and an athlete of my experience should have known better.

"At the end of the race my lungs were on fire and I felt as if they were bleeding. It hurt too much just breathing," he says. Three days later, when Koch had to drop out of another race after only a kilometer, he knew that he was in big trouble for the upcoming Olympic Games.

Although he realized that his lungs would prevent him from performing to his true abilities, Koch nevertheless went to Sarajevo for the Winter Games. For several days before the start of the competition, he didn't train, pampering himself as much as possible in the hope that he might at least make it through his 50-kilometer race. At that point he still refused to take any asthma medication and confided only to his coach about the pain in his lungs.

Koch's lungs improved only slightly as the Olympics went on. "They were very tender and I was breathing hard and wheezing heavily all during the Games," says Koch. "Surprisingly enough, though, I started out well in the fifty kilometer and was actually in the top ten for most of the race." Koch wasn't able to sustain his pace, however, and finished in seventeenth place.

Champion bicyclist Alexi Grewal is also a proponent of the non-pharmacological approach to EIB. Grewal, who signed a lucrative pro contract to race in Europe after capturing a gold medal in the road race at the 1984 Olympic Games, first took up cycling more from necessity than as a sport.

"I started when I was about eleven years old," Grewal says. "My family lived ten miles out of town, so to get in to visit my friends or go to a party, I needed a bike. I started competing that same year just as a hobby. I had no idea, of course, that it was going to turn into a career for me."

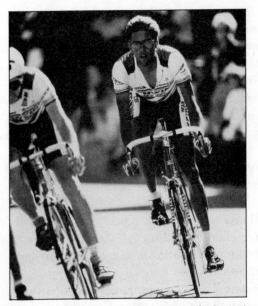

Alexi Grewal. (*Beth Schneider, copyright* © *1987*)

Cycling was fun for the Colorado native, but it certainly was never a matter of just getting on the saddle and starting to pedal for Alexi Grewal. Grewal, now twenty-eight, has EIB as well as allergenically based asthma. His EIB was first diagnosed in 1983, but he believes that his problems developed long before that time.

"I always had difficulty at the beginning of a race whenever I tried to go hard," Grewal recalls. "I would start gagging and I couldn't breathe properly. Whenever I inhaled, I couldn't take in a full breath. Then when I exhaled, I had difficulty getting a full breath out again."

Like Bill Koch, Grewal decided that medication wasn't for him. "I found after a while that it was a lot better for me to know my own body as best I could and to concentrate on getting in a good warm-up. Whenever I don't prepare well, my lungs just block up once the race begins." In contrast to Koch's warm-up, which lasts thirty to forty-five minutes, Grewal's warm-up period often lasts two hours. Most of us wish we had this amount of time for a complete workout!

Alexi Grewal's cycling preparations include making use of special breathing techniques to help keep his asthma in check. "I've been studying breathing for about three years," explains Grewal, who perfected his techniques with the help of Ian Jackson, a Texas athlete who has coined his yoga-based breathing approach "BreathPlay." (For more about Jackson and BreathPlay, see chapter 10.)

In addition to ragweed pollens, Grewal is bothered by air pollution when he's cycling. To get around this asthma trigger, he'll often try to hold his breath when he feels any constriction. "By putting my lungs under a lot of pressure, I can actually dilate the bronchial tubes and open them up," he says. "Whenever I'm in a race and I feel myself starting to gag, I'll hold my breath and the problem will usually pass."

Before the start of a race, when another athlete with asthma might use an inhaled bronchodilator, Alexi Grewal finds that it's helpful for him if he spends time meditating. "There are times when my asthma can be stress-related," he notes. "The more uptight and nervous I am before an event, the greater my chances of having an EIB attack. Meditation calms me down. I seek a quiet spot, collect my thoughts, and gradually relax myself."

Grewal, who also enjoys board sailing, cross-country skiing, and running when he's not on his bike, has these recommendations for people with asthma who are considering taking up a sport: "It's important right from the beginning that you become aware of what your limits are," he explains. "You'll know you've reached them when you first start experiencing some of the EIB symptoms like shortness of breath.

"No one can actually say what your limits are going to be because everyone's are so different," says Grewal. "But once you find your upper limit, the next time you go to exercise, push yourself gradually up to that limit and you'll see that the border can be pushed back a little further. Keep pushing, but don't go so hard that you bring on a major attack.

"The next time out you'll see that once again your limit has been extended a bit further. As you continue to exercise over the weeks, you'll be amazed to see that you keep pushing your limits bit by bit."

Grewal feels that the more you know about your asthma, the less you'll worry about it. "When you exercise you need to know that the asthma is there. But you also need to remember that you can learn to work within its limits."

Nonpharmacological Approach Questioned

While nonpharmacological methods are often used successfully by many world-class athletes in dealing with their EIB, they should not be used exclusive of medication, says William E. Pierson, M.D., who serves as codirector of the Exercise Induced Bronchospasm Project, a joint study sponsored by the U.S. Olympic Committee and the American Academy of Allergy and Immunology Sports Medicine Committee. Dr. Pierson tries to persuade athletes to consider the benefits of medication by pointing out the costs of the nonpharmacological approach.

"If an athlete has bronchospasm, he should use medication," says Dr. Pierson. "It's silly to try and work around potential bronchospasm through extra-long warm-ups and cool-downs. For me, this is like an athlete saying 'Should you change the flat tire on your car before driving it, or should you go out and drive until it goes totally flat?'

"Believe me," says Dr. Pierson, "it's not at all macho to compete with twenty percent to thirty percent airway obstruction from EIB just so you don't have to take the proper medication that could clear you right up."

As Dr. Pierson sees it, the major fault with the nonpharmacological approach in many instances is that it's rarely a complete solution to the problem of EIB. For an athlete in training or one who's in the midst of an important competition, one of the worst things that can happen is to develop EIB and be forced to cut back on practice or withdraw from competition.

Athletes train to be the very best they can be and are constantly pushing their limits. If they have to make Herculean efforts to avoid asthma during workouts and competition, then they are spending energy and time that could be much better used in their training or performance. "This doesn't have to happen if the athlete properly manages his asthma," says Dr. Pierson. "And asthma management means medication."

Dr. Roger Katz doesn't agree, because in his medical practice he has elite athletes who react quite differently from his other patients when it comes to medication. "The nonpharmacological approach won't totally eliminate the condition," says Katz. "Inhalers do a better job, without a doubt. But when dealing with elite athletes who refuse to take any kind of medications, you have to ask, 'What does this person really want?' Then you have to go and try to work that way for him."

For several years, Jackie Joyner-Kersee was one athlete who really did not want to take her asthma medication. But one day things changed dramatically for the worse and the twenty-six-year-old track star discovered for certain that without medication her athletic career would be a short one.

Olympic double gold medalist Jackie Joyner-Kersee, considered by experts to be the top female track-and-field athlete in the world, now takes medication for her asthma on a regular basis. There used to be a time, however, when she denied that she had asthma. On a cool morning at the UCLA track seven months prior to the 1988 summer Olympic Games in Seoul, her dreams of Olympic glory almost ended because of her denial and, more specifically, because of her unwillingness to follow her doctor's orders regarding medication.

"It was an easy training day," Jackie recalls. "We were running up the stadium steps and when I came off the last step I knew that something was really wrong with me. I couldn't breathe and I started getting really hot. I bent over, trying to catch my breath, but when I couldn't, I started to panic. I tried taking off my clothes in an effort to get in more air. I used my inhaler, but after a few puffs, I still didn't get any better. It really felt as if I was getting ready to die."

Jackie's husband, Bob Kersee, who's also her track coach, rushed her to the nearby hospital, where she was successfully treated in

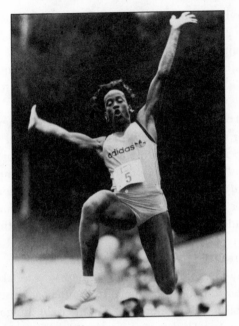

Jackie Joyner-Kersee.

the emergency room. Later, her physician, Dr. Katz, discovered that her theophylline blood concentration level was subnormal because she had not been taking her pills regularly as he'd instructed. That, combined with her exercising on a cold day when the grass in the stadium was being mowed, had been enough to trigger Jackie's severe asthma.

"When it comes to track, I'm in control," says Jackie. "I'm able to push myself to go fast but still not pull a muscle. I'm in control when I decide how far I want to jump or how fast I want to run the eight hundred meters. But I didn't have control when the asthma came over me that time, and it was scary."

The incident marked the first time in the four years since she had been diagnosed as having asthma that Jackie realized she could no longer take her medication whenever she felt like it. She knew she had to take all of it, as prescribed.

Although her doctor had prescribed both an albuterol inhaler and theophylline tablets, Jackie rarely took the tablets. "I never liked taking pills, not even aspirin," she explains. "I thought they would restrain me. Anyway, I asked myself, how can I be an athlete and have asthma? I tried getting by on the least amount of medicine possible. The albuterol inhaler worked for me, for a while at least."

Since that cold morning in Los Angeles, Jackie Joyner-Kersee has changed her ways. On a small piece of paper on her refrigerator, right next to a neat list of athletic goals she has set for herself, she has written: "Jackie: Take your medicine." This simple message and the vivid image of not being able to breathe are enough to make her heed her doctor's instructions. Her two gold medals are personal reminders of what can be achieved when asthma is dealt with properly.

"I finally realized that asthma is serious," she says. "I know that the only way I'm going to be able to compete is to take my medication regularly, both the pills and the inhaler. I also know that what I had been doing before was not the right thing to do."

Cheryl Durstein-Decker strikes a healthy balance between the pharmacological and nonpharmacological approaches to EIB management. Durstein-Decker is a full-time fitness consultant who also competes in triathlons whenever she has a chance. A typical triathlon might consist of a one-mile swim in choppy ocean waters, followed immediately by a bike ride of twenty-five to fifty miles, then by a run of ten or fifteen miles. A triathlon competition, depending on the distances, can take as little as one hour or as long as fifteen hours to complete.

The triathlon was never intended for anyone not in peak physical condition. As Durstein-Decker can attest, though, people with asthma need not shy away from the challenge. Triathlon training, a weekly mix of swimming, bicycling, and running, with some weight training thrown in to build strength and endurance, allows athletes to cross-train, that is, to work out regularly in several different sports. In addition to being more interesting, the major benefit of cross-training is that you can develop more speed, endurance, and strength from the multisport approach than you can from just one sport.

Durstein-Decker, now thirty-five, first developed asthma when she was twenty-eight, shortly after she began exercising in earnest for the first time in her life. "I decided right at the beginning that I was going to be a fighter, that I wasn't going to let my asthma act as a handicap to what I wanted out of life," Durstein-Decker recalls. "I was enjoying my exercise too much."

Durstein-Decker very deliberately sought out doctors who were knowledgeable, encouraging, and helpful when it came to assisting her pursue the active life-style she had chosen for herself. She recommends the same careful search to all sport-minded people with asthma. "The right doctors are definitely out there," she says. "If the physician you're seeing now isn't sympathetic enough or that well informed about exercise and asthma, then it's time to start looking for another doctor."

Durstein-Decker's doctors helped her work out an asthma medication program. Initially, this meant trying out several different types of drugs to see which worked best for her. She finally settled on one of the beta-agonists.

Today Durstein-Decker uses just one medication, terbutaline, both as an inhaler and in tablet form. A half hour before she's scheduled to compete in an Ironman-length triathlon (approximately 140 total miles), she takes a puff from the inhaler, then jogs or swims lightly as a warm-up. She finds that this warm-up period allows her to get the coughing and hacking out of the way and helps her to avoid any serious breathing problems during the race.

Just before the starting gun goes off, she takes another puff from the inhaler. Ninety minutes later she'll take her first tablet, repeating the dose every ninety minutes throughout the triathlon.

Durstein-Decker has complete confidence in medication, and thus has never hesitated to push herself all out in competition. She also has the confidence that comes from knowing that she's taken charge of her asthma and, as a result, is living life on her own terms.

"I feel that if I don't control my asthma, then it's going to control me," she says. "As long as I know that I'm the one who's in control because I'm dealing with the problem, then there's no reason why I can't go out and keep extending myself athletically."

This doesn't mean that Durstein-Decker is never bothered by her asthma. At the Ironman World Triathlon Championships in Hawaii, for example, she frequently has difficulty because of the intense heat. She's already competed in the Ironman (2.5-mile swim, 112-mile bike ride, 26.2-mile run) four times, and, while her swimming and cycling times have steadily improved, her marathon time has remained the same because the scorching Hawaiian sun causes her to become dehydrated by the time she's set to begin the running portion. That, in turn, dries out her airways and makes it hard for her to breathe properly.

"In 1985 I was dehydrated and had my slowest time," says Durstein-Decker. "If you had run by me and heard me hacking during the marathon, you'd probably have said, 'Pull that woman off the course before she dies.'" Durstein-Decker estimates that she drank gallons of water that day, force-feeding herself throughout the competition.

In addition to her medication, which she uses in training as well as in competition, Durstein-Decker employs several other methods to help manage her asthma. One is a set of special breathing exercises that focus on forcing the air out from her diaphragm and developing an easy, extended exhale rhythm. (For more detail, see chapter 10, "Breathing Exercises.")

Durstein-Decker also uses an array of mental training techniques to help her asthma and her athletic performance. The aim of these mind exercises is to be both physically and mentally primed for a good workout or competition. Although the impact of sport psychology is generally hard to measure, Durstein-Decker attributes a good portion of her success in managing her asthma and doing well in triathlons to the visualization techniques that she uses. "I would visualize even if I didn't have asthma," she says, "but I think that visualization becomes more important and valuable when you do have asthma."

Basically what Durstein-Decker does before a competition is close her eyes and visualize, actually picture herself, going through the motions she'll be taking in each particular event. For example, she sees herself breathing well in each event as she swims, cycles, and runs, in control of her body the whole while, taking medication when she needs it. Since asthma can be triggered by a hot, parched throat, she pictures herself sipping water every few minutes to keep her throat moist as she moves along the course. While training for a triathlon, Durstein-Decker will usually devote ten minutes to visualization for every hour of physical training that she'll put in that day.

"All in all," says Durstein-Decker, "it's important to realize that asthma doesn't have to be a roadblock that keeps you from what you want out of life. Not everyone, of course, can be a triathlete or compete in ultraendurance events. But everyone can take satisfaction in exercising, in pushing back your own mental and physical limits."

Personal satisfaction in exercise and sports competition comes from seeing what you can do, and in extending yourself to do more. "Look at it this way," says Durstein-Decker. "Asthma only gives you more limits to push back than anyone else. And once you do push those boundaries, your accomplishment will be that much more gratifying."

WHICH SPORT OR EXERCISE IS BEST?

People with asthma have competed at the world-class level in every sport. Still, some sports are less likely than others (but not always!) to trigger bronchospasm because they usually take place in warm, humid environments or indoors. For many EIB-prone exercisers, swimming, for example, turns out to be the near-perfect exercise, because swimmers are able to inhale humidified air that is right above the water. This seems to reduce effectively the cooling and drying of the airways, thereby limiting EIB episodes.

According to Dr. Roger Katz, the asthma and allergy specialist from Los Angeles, wrestling, weight training, baseball, football, and doubles tennis are also recreational as well as competitive sports that are good for people with EIB. "These sports are all carried out in relatively short bursts of energy," explains Dr. Katz. "And these short bursts aren't usually enough to stimulate the person's irritable airway."

In contrast, basketball, long-distance running, soccer, and cross-country skiing are, according to Dr. Katz, great EIB stimulators because of their nonstop nature and long-term intensity. Still, he says, this shouldn't preclude participation for people with EIB, as long as they work out a plan of management with their physician.

At one time, physicians automatically made swimmers out of their asthmatic patients. But now that asthma is better understood and excellent medications are available, it's better for people with asthma to pick a sport they enjoy and will stick with and then fit their management program to the sport.

MEDICATION FOR EIB

As you have seen, while there are some world-class athletes with EIB who are able to participate in their sports without taking medication, most physicians recommend that people who have EIB premedicate with an inhaled beta-agonist medication (such as Alupent, Metaprel, Proventil, or Ventolin) shortly before they exercise in order to prevent any bronchospasm. For those exercisers who develop bronchospasm infrequently, medication can be taken with a metered dose inhaler (MDI, also known as a "puffer" or an "inhaler") at the time of the flare-up during exercise in order to rid themselves of the symptoms.

The main EIB medications fall into three distinct drug groups: beta-adrenergic agents, cromolyn sodium, and theophylline. These medications are discussed in more detail in chapter 9, "Medication."

8

DOCTORS

THE RIGHT DOCTOR

In chapter 7, Cheryl Durstein-Decker, the triathlete, mentioned the importance of finding the right doctor if you have asthma and want to pursue a full, active life. I couldn't agree more; the point is worth repeating. All too often I meet people with asthma who tell me they would like to begin exercising and participating in sports but have always held back because their parents or physicians have cautioned against it. Even though this attitude has become harder to justify in recent years, there are still doctors who routinely dispense this kind of advice to their asthma patients. Some physicians are simply very set and rigid in their thinking; others have not stayed abreast of the new developments and discoveries in the asthma/exercise field. If you feel your doctor isn't listening to you, or can't or won't provide the type of help, understanding, and cooperation you need in order to live a life that includes exercise and sports, find another doctor.

Cheryl Durstein-Decker kept looking until she was satisfied that she had found someone she could work with. Given the right blend of medical supervision, support, and encouragement, she is now able to compete regularly in the triathlon, a sport that requires tremendous physical effort and endurance.

Joe Carabino, an All Ivy League basketball standout from Harvard who later went on to star in the European league, first had asthma when he was five years old. Luckily, his next-door neighbor was a doctor. An allergist was soon recommended and Joe went to him for the next five years. He took medication for his asthma and was given allergy shots four times a week. While his parents kiddingly called him "Wheezebag" and treated him no differently from their other five children, by the time Joe was ten, they saw that he wasn't getting much better and felt it was time to change doctors.

"We had been referred to my first doctor and we stayed with him," says Carabino, echoing a response of many people with asthma. Unfortunately for Carabino, his physician was overweight and didn't do any kind of sports himself. "My parents did some checking around and I switched to another doctor. It made a big difference in my life."

Carabino's new physician was a board-certified allergist and an expert in childhood asthma. He gave extensive exams and asked a battery of questions in order to get a good picture of Joe's health. "What I found to be so good about the new doctor was that he encouraged me do whatever I could in sports," says Carabino. Shortly after starting up with his new doctor, Carabino began playing basketball for his grade-school team and went on to lead it to four city championships.

George Murray, the leading wheelchair athlete, also credits his doctors for finally allowing him to take charge of his asthma and regain a measure of control in his life. Murray, who finished first in the 1978 Boston Marathon with a time of 2 hours, 26 minutes, developed asthma at the age of twenty when he left his native Maine to attend college at the University of Oklahoma.

"After the asthma was finally diagnosed, the doctors didn't do too much. I'd go see them periodically and they'd give me a pred- nisone treatment [prednisone is a corticosteroid medication that's administered either orally or by injection]. That would clean me up for a while, but sooner or later I would always be back for another one. In between treatments the only medication I took was an over-the-counter [OTC] bronchodilator—a lot of it. My doctors just never prescribed anything for me."

It was not until he moved to St. Petersburg, Florida, in the mid-1970s that Murray started to get a handle on his asthma. Two things made a big difference. "I began 'running' in my chair," Murray explains. "This provided me with a continual high level of aerobic exercise. I realized almost immediately that I enjoyed the speed and freedom and movement. The more I worked at my running, the better and faster I got. And it helped my lungs a lot.

"The other critical factor was that I finally got myself involved with a couple of asthma- and allergy-educated physicians at the University of South Florida. They put me on different kinds of medication [Theo-Dur and Vanceril] in a maintenance program which kept me symptom-free. Before this, I had only been treating the symptoms. I got rid of the OTC medications that I had been

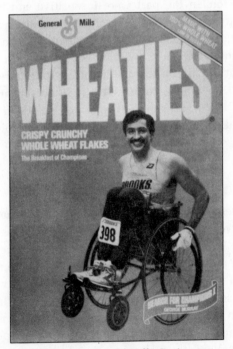

George Murray. (*General Mills, Inc.*)

using by the case and haven't used any since. With the new prescription medications I found that for the first time I could train as hard as I wanted and still remain symptom-free."

By 1981, Murray was feeling so well and had worked himself into such splendid physical condition that he "pushed" across the continent from Maine to California in his wheelchair. Each year now he competes in a full schedule of races, including several marathons. His personal best is 1 hour, 45 minutes, set in Boston in 1985. For all of his athletic achievements, Murray was selected to be on the Wheaties cereal box, an honor given only to a handful of athletes since the tradition started.

Murray continues to take his asthma medication without fail every morning and evening, whether or not he's experiencing any symptoms. If he does happen to get wheezy or begins coughing a lot, he goes in to see his doctor, who'll usually make an adjustment in the medication.

"Some doctors in the past were insensitive and tried to discourage me from exercising," Murray says. "But I now feel that they were ignorant, not just about asthma and how to treat it, but about what motivates an individual, and, most important, about what it is that constitutes the quality of life for different people."

As Cheryl Durstein-Decker says, the right doctors are definitely out there. If you're not geting all that you should from the one you're currently seeing, it may be time to start shopping around.

FINDING A DOCTOR

Once you decide that your current asthma care is inadequate for the life-style you've chosen, there are certain questions you should ask yourself. What type of doctor should I see? Where should I start to look? How will I know that he or she is the right doctor for me? What questions should I ask during the first visit?

There are several kinds of doctors who by their training and specialization are qualified to treat asthma. These include allergists, pulmonologists, internists, and, for children, pediatricians and pediatric allergists. In all cases, the physician you see should be board certified in his or her specialty. *Board certified* means that the physician has completed specialized training and received certification from an independent medical body that establishes qualifications and standards in the field.

A board-certified allergist is one who has been certified by the American Board of Allergy and Immunology in Philadelphia. Don't hesitate to ask your doctor or his or her receptionist about board certification. This is information you are entitled to.

After speaking with numerous athletes with asthma and medical professionals, I've found that a board-certified allergist is the physician of preference in most cases and the one most likely to be aware of the latest developments in the asthma/exercise field. You can obtain referrals for board-certified allergists in your area by contacting the following organizations:

American Academy of Allergy and Immunology
611 East Wells Street
Milwaukee, WI 53202
1-800-822-2762
414-272-6071

Asthma and Allergy Foundation of America
1717 Massachusetts Avenue, NW, Suite 305
Washington, DC 20036
1-800-7ASTHMA
202-265-0265

National Jewish Center for Immunology and
Respiratory Medicine
1400 Jackson Street
Denver, CO 80206
1-800-222-LUNG
303-388-4461

Your local chapter of the American Lung Association may also make referrals. This policy differs, however, from chapter to chapter.

To verify the status of a physician who is a board-certified allergist, contact:

American Board of Allergy and Immunology
3624 Market Street
Philadelphia, PA 19104
215-349-9466

You can also contact a sports-medicine clinic in your area to see if it can make referrals. For a good national directory that lists sports-medicine centers, send a self-addressed, stamped envelope to:

The Physician and Sportsmedicine Magazine
4530 West 77th Street
Minneapolis, MN 55435

or contact the magazine at 612-835-3222. The directory costs $15.

Another way to find a clinic is through your local medical association or the nearest medical school. Describe your situation and ask them to recommend an asthma specialist who treats athletes as a regular part of his or her practice. Who knows, you may even end up in the care of a physician who is also asthmatic and athletic!

When you have selected a doctor who has the qualifications and background you're looking for, make sure he or she is also someone you feel comfortable with, someone who listens and appreciates your input, someone who answers your questions fully and clearly without giving the impression that you're taking up his or her time. Most of all, make sure that your new doctor is willing to share your goals by working with you. The approach should be open, honest, and supportive.

VISITING THE DOCTOR

In evaluating a patient, the first step for the physician is to take time to talk with the patient about all clear-cut asthma symptoms and suspected asthma triggers, as well as life-style activities and expectations, including exercise programs and participation in sports. This information helps the doctor form a solid overall picture of events and triggers that might precipitate the patient's asthma.

As a patient, you should feel free and open with your physician and not just say what you think the doctor wants to hear. Be sure to note your earliest remembrances of discomfort and what you think may have brought on the trouble. Areas that should also be covered in this initial conversation include:

- Family history, including any incidences of respiratory trouble, allergies, sinus or nasal problems
- Your past medical history
- A complete listing of current symptoms, as well as runny nose and eyes, stomachache, unusual fatigue, and inactivity, especially in children
- Any medication you are currently taking, including over-the-counter medication

It's best to prepare for your first visit by writing down all pertinent information beforehand. With your information at hand, you won't be groping for dates and symptoms when the doctor asks for them, and you'll be less likely to forget something important. *The Asthma Organizer* ($17, Mothers of Asthmatics. Inc., 10875 Main Street, Suite 210, Fairfax, VA 22030, 703-385-4403) will help. This handy three-ring binder comes with asthma information as well as a daily home diary section, which is useful in tracking symptoms and early warning signals. There are also sections on peak-flow monitorings and coping with asthma in school.

In ensuing doctor visits, keep up a routine of having at least three questions to ask before you go to the office. Several studies have pointed out that patients are much more satisfied with the quality of their care when they have questions that are answered well by the doctor. This questioning builds a strong doctor-patient relationship.

"The confronting patient asks more questions," said Dr. Herman Feiffel, a Los Angeles psychologist. "They have an attitude that faces things squarely; they look directly at their illness, ask about it, and get specific information."

The major benefit of asking questions is that once you get information from your doctor you will be less anxious and have an increased sense of control over your asthma, both very important in proper asthma management.

LUNG-FUNCTION EXAM

Your physician needs to know how efficiently your lungs are currently functioning, that is, how well they're moving air in and out of your system. Does it take a little or a lot of effort for you to breathe? You can expect that he or she will administer a painless lung-function exam using a spirometer. This recording device measures the *amount* of air you're able to expel from your lungs, and the amount of *resistance* to airflow throughout your respiratory tract when you exhale.

If your doctor is having difficulty determining your asthma triggers, he or she may give you the spirometer test before and after having you inhale a bronchodilator, before and after exercise (which can be as simple as taking a lap around the office building), and before and after provocation with cold air, allergens, or methacholine (an inhaled histamine that can bring on a controlled asthma episode).

The spirometer test is very basic. After clipping your nostrils shut, the doctor will ask you to breathe into a mouthpiece, take a few breaths normally, and then inhale and exhale as much air from your lungs as possible. The results of the test are recorded on a graph. This measurement is called your forced air vital capacity (FVC). The maximum amount of inhaled air after a normal exhalation is called your inspiratory capacity, or IC.

Your results from the spirometer test will then be compared to medically predicted scores that are adjusted for your age, height, and sex. A score between 80 percent to 120 percent for your particular group is considered normal.

You may hear two numbers, your FVC and your FEV1. They stand for forced air vital capacity and forced expiratory vital capacity in one second, which indicates how much air you can move out of your lungs in one second as well as the degree of airway obstruction you might have. Obstruction is caused either by constriction of the air tubes by the smooth muscles surrounding them or by excess mucus clogging the airways, or, in many instances, by both.

COMMON PULMONARY FUNCTION TERMS

You may hear the following terms used by your doctor as he or she measures your lung function and capacity:

- *Total Lung Capacity (TLC)*: This is the amount of air in the lungs after a maximum inspiration, or how much air your lungs can currently hold.
- *Vital Capacity (VC)*: After you've taken in your deepest breath, this is the total amount of air that can be exhaled from the lungs, or, more basically, the total amount of air that you are able to move in and out of your lungs.
- *Tidal Volume (TV)*: This is the amount of air that would be inhaled and exhaled during a normal breath.
- *Inspiratory Capacity (IC)*: After taking a normal expiration, this is the maximum amount of air that can be inhaled.
- *Functional Residual Capacity (FRC)*: This is the amount of air left in the lungs after a normal expiration.
- *Residual Volume (RV)*: This is the amount of air left in the lungs after you've exhaled as much as you can.
- *Forced Air Vital Capacity (FVC)*: After you've taken your deepest breath, this is the greatest amount of air that can be exhaled the most forcefully.
- *Forced Expiratory Vital Capacity in One Second (FEV1)*: After you've inhaled as much as you can, this is the amount of air forcefully exhaled in one second.

PEAK-FLOW METERS

You can measure your breathing capacity at home by using a simple and inexpensive device called a peak-flow meter. This gadget measures how fast and hard you're able to exhale air from your lungs. It's a very useful instrument because flow rates may decrease several hours, sometimes even days, before an actual asthma episode occurs. The meter can serve as a warning you may be having problems long before you feel your first symptoms.

The peak-flow meter gives you a number indicating the velocity of air expelled in liters per second (l/sec.) or liters per minute (l/min.). You can compare the results with your predicted level and with your previous results. A drop of more than 10 percent below your normal readings may signal increased airflow resistance. You should talk to your doctor about it.

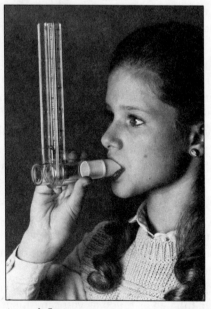

A peak-flow meter is an inexpensive home device used to measure current lung capacity. (*Assess*)

The reasons for the drop in the reading may be that your airways are constricted and swollen and mucus is accumulating; or that your particular medications may not be working as well as they usually do because "it's that time of the year" (pollen season); or that you may be coming down with a cold.

Using a peak-flow meter twice daily will provide you with early warning of asthma. It is also useful in teaching persons with asthma, especially children, how to become attuned to reading their bodily sensations. The person with asthma soon learns, "So this is what it feels like when I'm beginning to have an asthma episode," and then he or she can better manage the asthma.

There are many peak-flow meters currently available. They can be obtained from your doctor, your local pharmacy, or by ordering directly from the manufacturer. Be sure to follow the directions.

Remember that if you have a drop of between 10 percent and 40 percent over previous baseline readings, you are experiencing an asthma episode; a drop of 50 percent indicates you are in the danger zone. You and your physician should have established guidelines for what you should do next. If not, ask your doctor.

MEDICATION

New asthma medications have been developed that are very successful in controlling asthma symptoms. Most people with asthma don't need to take medication on a daily basis, but when asthma does flare, properly prescribed drugs (based on a patient's condition and the effectiveness of a particular drug in combating asthma) will bring it under control quickly and with limited, if any, side effects. Once again, be sure to consult with your doctor in the use of drugs for asthma.

There are five types of medication that doctors usually prescribe for asthma: beta-adrenergic agents, theophylline, cromolyn sodium, corticosteroids, and anticholinergics.

BETA-ADRENERGIC AGENTS

Beta-adrenergic agents, or beta-agonists as they are frequently called, are bronchodilators. This means that they work by relaxing the smooth bronchial muscles surrounding the airways, thus keeping them from constricting. These adrenalinelike medications include albuterol (Proventil, Ventolin), terbutaline (Brethaire), bitolterol (Tornalate), pirbuterol (Maxair), and metaproterenol (Alupent, Metaprel), and are extremely effective in relieving acute or sudden asthma symptoms. They can be taken either orally (in liquid or tablet form) or, more commonly, by inhalation. When inhaled, they provide the quickest relief with little effect on the heart or blood circulation.

Inhaled beta-agonists are especially effective during acute episodes and in preventing exercise-induced bronchospasm (EIB). Taken fifteen to twenty minutes before starting exercise, two puffs from an inhaler are usually enough for four hours of protection. Side effects of the metered-dose inhaled medications are almost nonexistent, although some people may experience headache, nervousness, and body tremors. Most beta-agonists are approved for use in national and international sports competitions and in many cases are the only medication an athlete with asthma uses.

THEOPHYLLINE

Theophylline is a bronchodilator that works by relaxing the smooth muscles of the air passages, thereby opening up the bronchial tubes. Theophylline also prevents the release of mediators (such as histamines) from the mast cells. It's currently the most widely prescribed medication for the treatment of chronic and severe asthma and is available under a number of brand names in liquid, capsule, and tablet form.

Although it is the most widely prescribed medication for chronic asthma, theophylline has varied side effects, such as insomnia, diarrhea, and stomach cramps, that have led many physicians to switch to albuterol as the first drug of choice. If albuterol proves to be ineffective, the patient may be switched to cromolyn sodium, followed by a daily dose of inhaled steroids if the cromolyn fails as well. Then comes theophylline. If you have been recently diagnosed as having asthma and your physician wants to start you on a long-term theophylline regime, it's not inappropriate to ask him or her why it's not prudent to try the other medications first.

Theophylline can be tricky to use. If you're athletic and have EIB, you may have to schedule your theophylline intake so that it reaches its peak effectiveness at the time that you plan to exercise or compete. In lengthy workouts or endurance-type competitions, however, that peak time can often be difficult to pinpoint. To make matters more difficult, in sports in which there is excessive body water lost through perspiration, such as cross-country or marathon running, football or basketball, therapeutic blood levels of the-ophylline can be adversely affected and complications can set in, such as headache, nausea, or overall jitters.

When you take theophylline on a daily basis, it's important that your blood levels be monitored regularly to make sure you are receiving a proper dose consistent with your age, weight, and de-gree of asthma severity. Doctors' opinions vary on how often you should have your blood tested. Some physicians recommend that you be tested every six months, some say every four months. In any case, if you feel that your asthma symptoms are getting worse, consult your physician.

Theophylline blood tests can be performed in a well-equipped physician's office, usually with the blood taken from a prick of the finger. Results are usually ready in fifteen to twenty minutes. Ther-apeutic theophylline levels range from ten to twenty micrograms per milliliter of blood. Anything above or below this range often means the theophylline dose must be changed. Changing your the-ophylline dosage yourself without consulting your physician is not advised. Theophylline is a tricky medication, one with a fine line between effectiveness and toxicity.

CROMOLYN SODIUM

Cromolyn sodium is a preventive medication that works by keeping mast cells in the lungs from releasing mediators (such as histamine) in the presence of allergens or irritants, thus preventing the airways from closing. Unlike the beta-agonists, cromolyn is not very effec-tive in reversing or relieving an acute asthma episode.

Many athletes don't like using cromolyn because it must be taken every day. The good news, however, is that it has virtually no side effects. For some people, cromolyn may have to be taken for several weeks before it becomes effective. For this reason, athletes who have important competitions coming up in areas problematic for people with asthma begin taking cromolyn three to four weeks before their competition.

Cromolyn (Intal) has proved effective in preventing EIB. Approximately 50 percent of those who premedicate regularly thirty to forty-five minutes before exercising develop no symptoms.

CORTICOSTEROIDS

If a person's asthma can't be controlled by beta-agonists, theophylline, or cromolyn sodium, the physician will then prescribe corticosteroids. These powerful drugs are derived from cortisone and can be used effectively to prevent chronic asthma symptoms as well as fight acute episodes. In cases of status asthmaticus, an asthma episode that lasts more than twenty-four hours with an accompanying risk of death from respiratory failure or exhaustion, the antiinflammatory properties of corticosteroids will often bring the asthma under control quickly.

Corticosteroids, which are not normally used in the prevention or treatment of EIB, should not be confused with anabolic steroids. These drugs, whose use is banned in all international competition, are used by some unethical athletes to help build up muscle mass and increase strength.

Corticosteroids are available in an inhaled form, and many doctors are now using them as the first line of treatment of asthma. Inhaled steroids, also known as topical steroids, are often taken after using a bronchodilator to help reduce late-phase airway inflammation. In aerosol form, this medication goes directly to the airways, is minimally absorbed by the body, and therefore doesn't produce the side effects of steroids taken orally. However, it is recommended that you have a drink of water after using inhaled steroids to prevent throat infections and hoarseness. Inhaled forms include flunisolide (AeroBid), beclomethasone (Beclovent, Vanceril), and triamcinolone (Azmacort).

When taken orally in pill form over long periods of time, corticosteroids can have potentially dangerous side effects, which include growth suppression, weight gain, hypertension, osteoporosis, cataracts, muscle weakness, mood swings, and facial swelling. Patients with acute asthma are often given steroids as a lifesaving measure and must then be closely monitored by their physicians. Frequently used oral corticosteroids include prednisone, methylprednisolone, and prednisolone.

ANTICHOLINERGICS

A class of drugs relatively new to the United States, but used successfully in Europe and Canada for several years for the treatment of chronic bronchitis, is the anticholinergic. Ipratropium bromide (Atrovent) is a bronchodilator that's administered with an inhaler, and it's been found to be quite successful in reducing mucus production and coughing. Unlike albuterol, which has bronchodilating effects in ten to fifteen minutes, anticholinergics may take one to two hours before they're effective. For this reason, this medication is recommended for use along with albuterol, to relieve chronic cough and other symptoms of bronchitis, and not as a primary asthma medication. Still, asthma specialists are hoping for good results with the drug as more people begin to use it.

OVER-THE-COUNTER MEDICATIONS

In addition to the numerous prescription medications, there are just as many over-the-counter medications (OTCs) that are available without prescription at your local pharmacy. Some are effective in treating *mild* and *infrequent* cases of asthma. OTCs are bronchodilators usually containing ephedrine or epinephrine, another name for adrenaline. They are available in inhaler or tablet form and can be very helpful when asthma flares up and you don't have your prescription medication. Once, in the middle of a press interview, Jackie Joyner-Kersee, the 1988 Olympic double gold medalist, started to wheeze and found it hard to breathe. To her dismay, when she went to her pocketbook, she found that she'd forgotten her prescription medication. Her husband ran to a nearby pharmacy and came back with an OTC for Jackie to use. Fifteen minutes later she was feeling better and called her physician to report to him. Always consult with your physician before using an OTC medication.

As Jackie Joyner-Kersee found out, OTC medications can be helpful for temporary (albeit very short-term) relief of asthma symptoms. Unfortunately, OTCs often lull users into the mistaken notion that their asthma is under control and that they are doing all they can to manage it. In many cases, proper treatment of underlying asthma problems and causes may be delayed or ignored altogether.

The other danger of OTC medications is that they can be overused because their effectiveness is of such short duration (usually fifteen minutes). Overuse can result in serious side effects such as nausea, nervousness, and heart palpitations, and may lead to dangerous health problems. Use OTC medication only in temporary emergency situations and visit your doctor soon after for a better asthma management program.

MEDICINE CAUTIONS

1. Know your medication by generic name, brand name, and dosage, and know when to take it.

2. Know the usual and unusual side effects of your medicines.

3. Keep an up-to-date, clearly written list of your current medicines, schedule, and dose. One copy should be with a member of the family or a friend and another copy in your wallet or car.

4. Call your doctor for a refill of your medicine if it is three-fourths empty.

5. Keep extra medicine in handy places such as the glove compartment of your car, your lunch box, briefcase, office desk, locker, and vacation home so you won't be caught

without it. Make sure medications are in child-proof containers.

6. Know the expiration date of your medicine. Ask your pharmacist to write it on the bottle.

7. Learn exactly how to use your inhaler. Bring it along when you visit your doctor so he or she can observe how you use it.

8. Don't overuse your inhaler.

9. Never take more medicine than is prescribed.

10. Before taking your medicine, be sure to read its label.

11. Color-code your medicine bottles if you are taking two or more different tablets or capsules. This is especially helpful for children.

12. Keep a checklist if you are taking many medicines regularly. Avoid taking double doses or forgetting a dose.

13. Don't take over-the-counter medicine or any new medicine without consulting your doctor. Many medications can interfere with the effect of theophylline.

SOURCE: Adapted from *Asthma Today* newsletter, 412 State Street, Bangor, ME 04401

Asthma Medications

Generic Name	Brand	How Taken
BETA-ADRENERGIC AGENTS		
Albuterol	Proventil, Ventolin	Inhaler, syrup, tablet, solution, rotahaler
Terbutaline	Brethaire, Brethine, Bricanyl	Inhaler, tablet, injection, solution
Bitolterol	Tornalate	Inhaler
Pirbuterol	Maxair	Inhaler

Generic Name	Brand	How Taken
Metaproterenol	Alupent, Metaprel	Inhaler, tablet, solution, syrup

CROMOLYN SODIUM

Cromolyn	Intal	Powder, solution, inhaler

CORTICOSTEROIDS

Prednisone	Deltasone, Liquid Pred	Tablet, syrup
Beclomethasone	Beclovent, Vanceril	Inhaler
Flunisolide	AeroBid	Inhaler
Triamcinolone	Azmacort	Inhaler with spacer

ANTICHOLINERGIC

Ipratropium bromide	Atrovent	Inhaler

THEOPHYLLINE

Theophylline comes in liquid, tablet, or capsule form. Brand names include: Accurbron, Aerolate, Aquaphyllin, Asbron, Azpan, Brondecon, Bronkodyl, Choledyl, Constant-T, Dilor, Duraphyl, Elixophyllin, Lodrane, Lufyllin, Marax, Mersalyl-Theophylline, Mudrane, Primatene Tablet, Quadrinal, Quibron, Respbid, Slo-bid, Slo-Phyllin, Somophyllin, Sustaire, Synophylate, Tedral, Theobid, Theoclear, Theo-Dur, Theofedral, Theolair, Theon Syrup, Theo-Organidin, Theophylline Oral, Theospan-SR, Theostat 80 Syrup, Theo-24, Theovent, Uniphyl.

BANNED DRUGS

Olympic, National Collegiate Athletic Association (NCAA), and international sports rules permit athletes with asthma to use many different asthma medications as long as their physicians notify the appropriate sport governing board. Currently, inhaled albuterol, cromolyn sodium, terbutaline, and theophylline are all approved medications. Inhaled epinephrine (adrenaline) and ephedrine are banned substances because of their stimulating effect on the body's nervous system.

At the 1988 Olympic Games in Seoul, South Korea, Canadian sprinter Ben Johnson was stripped of his gold medal in the 100-meter dash because traces of anabolic steroids, a muscle-building drug, were found in his mandatory urine sample. When the story was first reported, many people were reminded of another drug incident sixteen years earlier at the 1972 Games in Munich. At that time, Rick DeMont, a sixteen-year-old high school swimmer from San Rafael, California, had to forfeit the gold medal he had just won in the 400-meter freestyle. In addition, DeMont was barred from competing in the 1,500-meter freestyle, his best event, and was asked to leave the Olympic Village.

What had the teenager done to warrant such harsh treatment? DeMont, it was revealed, had violated International Olympic Committee (IOC) drug rules. Infinitesimal traces of ephedrine, an adrenalinelike stimulant banned by the IOC, had turned up in the urine sample DeMont was required to submit after his victory in the 400-meter freestyle. Ephedrine, in very small quantities, is one of the ingredients in Marax, an asthma medication commonly prescribed by physicians at the time but currently no longer in widespread use.

DeMont had been taking Marax for years to treat his severe asthma and allergies and, in compliance with IOC regulations, had been careful to inform the American Olympic team doctors about the medication and his asthmatic condition. However, the doctors had failed to pass this information to the IOC's medical board for clearance, and, as a result, DeMont eventually suffered the consequences.

Unlike athletes who knowingly use anabolic steroids, Rick DeMont had never intended to deceive anyone or gain an unfair advantage over his competitors. In DeMont's case, the ephedrine may actually have been a disadvantage because of the nervousness and tension that it causes. The teenager had simply been caught up in a set of circumstances that were entirely beyond his control. To this day, it is still painful for DeMont to think about the incident and the manner in which it was handled. "I don't want to be remembered as the famous gold medal loser," he says.

DeMont's troubles with asthma date back to long before the '72 Games. At the age of two he developed extremely bad allergies and eczema and a year later was diagnosed for asthma. Before his condition became stabilized with medication, there were numerous trips to the hospital emergency room for adrenaline injections to quell his asthma. By the age of four, he was visiting the doctor twice a week for allergy shots in both arms. Throughout his early childhood, DeMont remembers being awakened in the middle of the night, every night, to take a pill of some sort. Besides Marax, DeMont was also taking Sudafed, Actifed, and Benadryl, all of which were prescription medications at the time.

Rick's mother became quite adept at handling the special needs and demands required just to get Rick through the day without a major episode. "He was allergic to just about everything. We always had to be so careful, " Mrs. DeMont recalls. "Anything could set him off—pollen, dust, trees, grasses, animal hair, chocolate, wheat, peanuts, and milk. Whenever he ate wheat, his stomach would cramp and bloat up. When he was a child, his abdomen was often huge, and he'd get a lot of teasing about it from the other kids."

Mrs. DeMont recalls that she was constantly looking for new ways to make Rick's home environment "safer" for him, especially his bedroom. "He had a great deal of trouble at night with his wheezing and mucus," says Mrs. DeMont. "We had humidifiers in the room, but the coughing got so bad sometimes that he couldn't catch his breath. I had to put a stack of books at the foot of his bed to raise it so that his head would be lower than his feet. That helped a little and he was able to breathe easier."

Still, Mrs. DeMont never discouraged Rick from going out and playing with the other children in the neighborhood. "I never tried to pamper Rick or restrict his activity or set him apart from other kids in a way that might make him feel that he was different," says Mrs. DeMont. "There were many times when he looked very pale and sickly with big reddish circles under his eyes. And he was prone to flus and infections. But I just felt it was important not to baby him. I did all I could not to play up the asthma too much."

Rick began swimming at the age of seven. His allergist recommended that he take up the sport because he believed it would be good for his lungs. It wasn't long before Rick was spending most of his time at the pool after school and on weekends. Swimming was not only the right exercise for his asthma, but an activity that seemed to suit him temperamentally as well. He could never get enough of it.

Rick progressed rapidly as a swimmer and was soon competing in local and state meets, where he dominated in the middle-distance events. By the time he finished his junior year of high school in June 1972, he had been named All-American three times and had set a new American mark in the 400-meter freestyle. At the Olympic trials in Chicago that summer, he broke the world record for the 1,500-meter freestyle and headed into the Olympics brimming with confidence and high expectations. At just sixteen years of age he seemed to have nearly limitless potential. And because his success had come despite his asthma, it was that much more meaningful to him. In Munich, however, everything came to a shattering and heartbreaking end.

The night before he was to swim in the 400-meter free final, Rick woke up coughing, wheezing, and unable to breathe. He didn't know what had triggered this episode, but he immediately began taking his asthma medication. Several days before, in accordance with IOC regulations, he had filled out a medical questionnaire and notified the USA team doctors of exactly which prescription medications he used for his asthma. These included some items— such as Marax, Sudafed, and Actifed—that were banned by the IOC. Rick had assumed (perhaps too trustingly) that since none of the American doctors had said anything to him, his list of medications had been cleared by the IOC and it was all right to take them.

By the time of the 400-meter free final, Rick had taken four doses of asthma medication over the previous twenty-four hours. He swam the 400 that day in his best time ever, eclipsing his old mark by nine-tenths of a second and winning the race by one-hundredth of a second, surging past the second-place finisher just near the wall.

Moments later, as he stood on the awards podium and had the gold medal placed around his neck, he was given a tremendous standing ovation by the crowd, and he felt himself choking with pride and emotion. "I couldn't believe that I had actually done it," Rick remembers. "There I was at the top of the world and everyone was watching. I was tingling at the moment. I had goose bumps. I nearly broke down and cried, I was so happy."

Two days later the fairy tale started to unravel. One of the managers of the swimming team showed up at Rick's quarters in the Olympic Village that morning and asked to see the medications he had been using. Rick was told that this was strictly a formality since he had already turned in a urine sample after his 400-meter victory.

The next day, after swimming a 1,500-meter heat and qualifying for the final, Rick was summoned to appear before the IOC rules committee. "I was totally scared," Rick recalls. "I was like a little kid in there, standing alone before all these important people from all over the world. After a while I could sense, just from the questions they asked, that some of them had already made up their minds about me. Several of them said they doubted that I even had asthma. It was hard for me to believe this, after all I had gone through with it. They asked me to describe an asthma attack and then to act one out for them. I didn't know what to do. How do you act out something like this?"

The next afternoon, as he paced nervously in the entrants' waiting room trying to rid his mind of distractions and focus on the 1,500-meter final just minutes away, he heard his name broadcast over the loudspeakers. A chill shot through him, and he knew at once that something terrible was going to happen. The steely voice traveling over the loudspeakers announced that Rick DeMont of the United States had been disqualified from the upcoming race.

Rick was devastated. Not only was he barred from swimming in the 1,500, he was also asked to return his gold medal, and then ignominiously expelled from the Olympics. In less than a week he had gone from being on the top of the world to being disgraced in front of it.

Mrs. DeMont feels that Rick has never really gotten over the incident even after all these years. "He's buried it someplace, but it will always be there," she says. "Rick was completely disillusioned by it. He just couldn't believe that the adult world could ever have treated him that way."

After the Olympics, Rick took some time off to recover from the heartache of Munich. A few months later he returned to training, coming back in 1973 to have one of the finest years in his career. At the world swimming championships in Belgrade, Yugoslavia, that season, he became the first person to break the mythical four-minute barrier in the 400-meter freestyle, a feat that people said could never be done. Soon after this triumph he was named Swimmer of the Year.

Rick is now retired from active competition and resides in Tucson, Arizona, where he devotes much of his time to his artwork. He also coaches and teaches swimming to children. Whenever he finds pupils who have asthma, he is very direct and encouraging in the advice he offers. "The first thing I tell them is not to let asthma hold them back from swimming or anything else in this life. See your doctor and take your medication the way you should. Then do whatever it is, whatever sport that you want. And remember that it's not asthma that will limit you or keep you from fulfilling your dreams. Only you can create your own limits."

$\backslash 1_0$

BREATHING EXERCISES

If you needed one catchall phrase to characterize the basic problem that all people with asthma face, you might choose "difficulty in breathing." Breathing, a natural process that happens easily and automatically for most people, turns into effort and struggle for people with asthma. We become hungry and desperate for air, and no one who has not experienced that sensation can quite understand what it feels like.

Nonasthmatics never have to think twice about their breathing or the functioning of their lungs. But for those of us with twitchy airways, there are moments when we are forced to spend all our time thinking just about breathing. Naturally, one of the things we often talk about is how to breathe better. As I travel around the country and speak to people with asthma or parents of asthmatics, I am frequently asked what we can do to improve our lungs and make them more efficient. First, I always encourage people to begin exercising to get themselves more aerobically fit. I often tell them about many of the athletes with asthma whose stories appear in this book. In addition, I recommend that they start practicing a few simple breathing exercises on a regular basis.

People rarely use their lungs at full capacity when breathing, because the portion that we do use is usually sufficient to get us

139

through our round of daily activities. Since we seldom call upon that unused reserve (approximately one-quarter to one-third our total lung capacity), it remains undeveloped. For people with asthma, tapping into this storehouse can prove beneficial.

The major benefit of breathing exercises is that they can teach you to breathe more fully, strengthening and expanding your lungs as oxygen is carried to underutilized lung tissue, in turn reducing the frequency and severity of asthma. Breathing exercises can also be used during asthma to help you relax and ride out the worst episode.

Karin Smith, a four-time Olympian in the javelin throw, has been taking asthma medication since 1984, when she was first diagnosed as having EIB and allergy-induced asthma. She's not happy about using the medication because it often gives her the shakes, and also because she considers medicine a passive approach to dealing with her health. So she does breathing exercises, which have been a great help.

"Finally taking an active part in my treatment and getting control of my breathing means a lot to me," says Smith, who was first taught how to breathe differently (from her diaphragm) several years ago by her Athletics West track-team sport psychologist, Dr. Scott Pengelly. "Before, when I couldn't get in enough air I would start to panic, which made my asthma much worse. However, after I started with the breathing exercises, this problem has been virtually eliminated."

DIAPHRAGMATIC BREATHING

The first type of breathing exercise I recommend is one that gets the diaphragm (a large muscle just beneath the lungs and above the abdomen) more fully involved in the act of breathing. As the lungs fill when you inhale, the diaphragm moves downward. As the lungs empty when you exhale, the diaphragm moves upward. By concentrating on your diaphragm as you breathe, you can allow the lungs to expand more fully during inhalation and empty more completely during exhalation.

The easiest way to practice diaphragmatic breathing is to sit, stand, or lie on your back and hold the palm of your hand against your stomach between your navel and rib cage. Breathe in deeply. If you are using your diaphragm to breathe, your stomach will push out against your hand. Now, exhale, and you should be able to feel your stomach go down as your hand moves in toward your stomach. Practice this several times a day for a few minutes at a time.

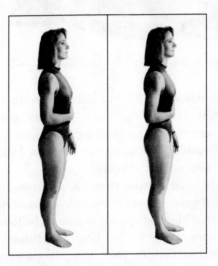

Once you're comfortable with this exercise, and breathing from the diaphragm becomes a little more natural for you, you may want to enhance the exercise by introducing a count for each of the two phases of the breath cycle. Begin by inhaling to a count of 4—at each count take in a little air so that by the 4 count your lungs are fully inflated—and exhaling to a count of 8. Again, let the air out in short stages until it's all expelled by the 8 count.

Practice this for several days, then begin to raise the exhale count slowly, keeping the inhale count at 4. Keep doing this, concentrating on letting the air out very slowly. See how high you can go on the exhale count until you feel you have no more air left to expel.

A variation on the diaphragmatic breathing exercise is to lie on your back and place about five pounds of weights on your diaphragm. A five-pound barbell plate, a bag of rice, a few books, or two bricks will do nicely. Suck in deeply with your diaphragm and exhale slowly as before. Repeat the exercise ten to twenty times.

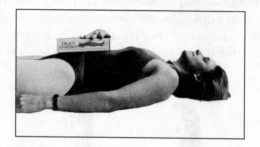

Dr. Leo Leonidas, the children's asthma specialist from Bangor, Maine, who edits the *Asthma Today* monthly newsletter, offers the following exercise for practicing diaphragmatic breathing, as well as some valuable suggestions on what to do if you feel yourself starting to have an asthma episode.

Put your right hand on your stomach, right over your belly button. Put your left hand on your chest, right in the center. Now, close your eyes and start blowing up a big imaginary balloon. Really push the air out of your lungs into this imaginary balloon. Push hard.

Each time that you empty your lungs, take a very deep breath and really fill up your lungs.

When you breathe in, see which hand moves first. It should be your right hand, the one on your belly. Your left hand shouldn't move at all, or at least not as much as your right hand.

When you start having trouble breathing during asthma, try to concentrate on breathing very slowly and evenly. Don't panic and start gasping for breath. Just sit still for a moment, let your shoulders droop a little, and concentrate on taking slow, deep breaths.

Visualize pulling the air all the way up your legs into your chest. Pull the air all the way up from your legs and into your lungs.

When you breathe out, pretend that you're pushing the air all the way back down your legs.

It's important that you give yourself a lot of time to breathe. Every time you fill your lungs up with air, let the air stay there for a couple of seconds. Then as you breathe out, you'll feel your legs begin to get heavy as you become calm and quiet.

OTHER BREATHING EXERCISES

In addition to the diaphragmatic breathing exercises described, I've found other exercises to be very effective in increasing overall lung capacity. They will help you expand your rib cage and allow you to breathe more deeply. Perform them each day, but especially during your pre-exercise warm-up. Perform each of the four exercises standing up with your feet shoulder-width apart, and repeat each exercise ten times.

1. With knees slightly bent, lift your arms over your head while inhaling as deeply as possible. Stretch and reach for the sky, looking up without arching your back. Try to feel your rib cage move away from your spine.

2. Bend over as far as feels comfortable while exhaling, hands pointed toward your feet. Don't force the stretch. It should feel good, not painful. Exhale all the way. Stand up slowly while inhaling deeply.

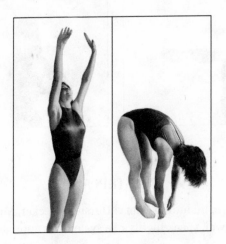

3. With knees slightly bent, arms straight out from your sides and parallel to the ground, inhale as slowly and deeply as possible. Exhale while twisting as far as possible to the right. Let your body positions help you exhale and inhale. As you return to face forward, inhale slowly. Twist to the left, exhaling as you make the move; inhale as you return to face forward.

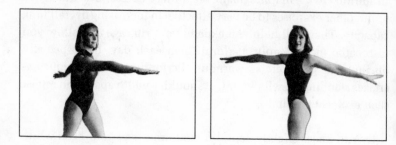

4. With knees slightly bent, hands together directly in front of you and arms parallel to the ground, exhale. While bringing your hands back to the sides of your body, elbows tucked in and behind you, inhale slowly. See how far you can expand your rib cage.

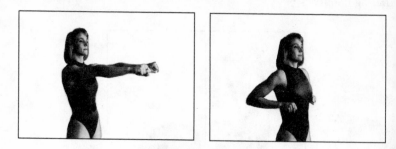

BREATHPLAY

Several athletes, including Cheryl Durstein-Decker, Mike Gminski, and Alexi Grewal, speak highly of a systematic approach to breathing developed by Ian Jackson, the fitness trainer and accomplished triathlete from Texas.

Jackson, who studied yoga for many years, has drawn heavily upon it for his breathing techniques. He calls his breathing method BreathPlay and says that with some practice you can "teach yourself how to use the ceaseless flow of air within to make your life work better." He has written a book on the subject called *The BreathPlay Approach to Whole Life Fitness* (Garden City, N.Y.: Doubleday, 1986).

The essence of Jackson's system is to teach us to concentrate on exhalation and make it the active half of the breathing process— vacate the lungs with a final contraction of the diaphragm—while inhalation becomes the passive half. Following Jackson's instructions, breathing out is done in steps of your own choosing, rather than in one steady stream of air. Concentrate on your belly and, in steps, make it go as flat as possible. Then let your lungs fill up the same way, one step at a time. Jackson believes that this staged breathing will help improve performance, block out pain, and reduce fatigue. He also feels that this active outbreath can be of great benefit for people with asthma.

In essence, when using Jackson's BreathPlay you are pushing out the *old* air and letting in the *new* air. Jackson likens his breathing techniques to squeezing the air out of a ball held tightly in your fist. Release the ball and the air is automatically sucked back in. You can do the same thing with your stomach, says Jackson. The trick is to use your abdominal muscles to expel the air by pulling them tight. When you release the muscles, your belly expands once again, sucking in air.

This sounds more complicated in the telling than it is in practice. Don't be scared away! Jackson provides a whole series of well-thought-out games and exercises for practicing each of the points in his breathing system, as well as numerous applications for the BreathPlay method in all major aerobic sports. His book is filled with many lively case histories, which give it a very personal touch despite the theoretical groundwork.

Although Jackson doesn't specifically address his book to people with asthma, he has worked with world-class asthmatic athletes in the past and has counseled many others at the BreathPlay clinics he gives around the country. Many athletes who have experimented with Jackson's theories speak of increased stamina and power, as well as better breathing. Alexi Grewal, the 1984 gold medalist in cycling, has asthma and credits Jackson's breathing techniques for helping him succeed as an athlete despite his asthma.

Cheryl-Durstein Decker, the triathlete, applies Jackson's techniques to her workouts and races and has found that she can breathe easier and has less trouble with her asthma. "Jackson teaches asthmatics that instead of concentrating on taking air in, they should focus on the exhale portion of their breathing," Durstein-Decker says. "If we concentrate on getting the air out, new air will come back in naturally."

In her workouts, Durstein-Decker strives for a forceful and rhythmic exhale as she breathes from her diaphragm. "When I'm on my bike, I use an exhale rhythm every other pedal stroke," she said. "When I'm running, I'll exhale for every five steps and inhale for three, exhale for five, inhale for three, and so on.

"There's a long count for the exhale and a shorter count for the inhale, when I just let the air come back in. Because I'm only thinking about pushing the air out, I tend to worry less about whether enough air is going to enter. After a while, that constant struggling and straining for oxygen begins to decrease."

Several years ago, Mike Gminski, the center for the Philadelphia 76ers basketball team, worked with a breathing coach in New Jersey who introduced him to Jackson's BreathPlay system. Gminski feels the breathing lessons have helped him a great deal. "You learn that the outbreath becomes active and the inbreath becomes passive," Gminski says. "Most people would think it's the other way around. That's because when we take a deep breath, we have a tendency to consciously raise our shoulders, so that we fill only the top third of our lungs. But if you compress your abdomen and blow air out on your outbreath, then your whole lung will fill back up with air once you release the outbreath. The amount of oxygen that you can take in becomes much greater as well."

Gminski uses short, twenty-to-thirty-minute walks in his free time to practice his breathing exercises. By concentrating on his

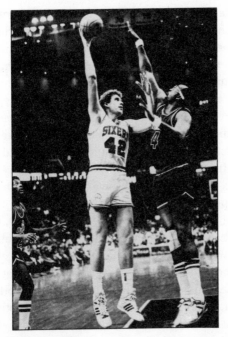

Mike Gminski.

breathing techniques, he's finding that they're gradually becoming a reflex for him. Although he can't give much thought to breathing techniques when he's caught up in the flow of an NBA game, he does practice breathing while sitting on the bench waiting to get back in the game. "In this way I'm able to aerate myself while watching the game," says Gminski. "It allows me to get a lot more fresh oxygen a lot quicker. That's important because once I'm back in the game, I'll need it."

Ian Jackson believes that his breathing techniques help create a relaxed mood, which can then help prevent "suffocation anxiety," the feeling that comes when you start gasping for air during a hard workout or when you have asthma. Jackson has his own story about the effectiveness of BreathPlay; he told me of a woman with asthma who had attended one of the BreathPlay clinics he gave at a fitness retreat in the Virgin Islands one summer.

"The retreat was at a camp built into the densely wooded slopes surrounding a bay," said Jackson. "The cabins were like tree houses, and they were connected by a network of raised wooden walkways. There were lots of stairs to climb, especially the long flights that went all the way down to the beach. It wasn't an ideal setting for someone with breathing difficulties.

"Jean came to my first BreathPlay session rather depressed. She was frustrated at being in such a paradise and yet in such deep anxiety over not being able to get in enough air. She was unable to relax and enjoy herself, and she moved slowly and awkwardly, frequently using her inhaler to open her air passages.

"I took note of her inhaler and suggested that she try instead an 'exhaler perspective.' Instead of working at getting air in, I said, try working at getting it out. The more you push out, the more air returns to fill the emptiness. Pushing air out gives a feeling of power and control, whereas trying to suck air in triggers anxiety about not getting enough. I had her play with pushing her air out and letting it back in, instead of the standard in-out method. She remarked, as did others, that it felt unnatural to breathe the way I suggested, but that it felt relaxing nevertheless. She was willing to give it a try. In making this change, Jean didn't have to do any special exercise; she simply worked on pushing her air out by pulling her belly back.

"At the next class, Jean reported that she was still carrying her inhaler but that she no longer used it as often. Her only complaint was that the active outbreathing was making her belly muscles sore. I pointed out that she was not only breathing better but whittling her waistline as well.

"By the third class Jean's worries about not being able to enjoy the Caribbean paradise were a thing of the past and she was leaving her inhaler back in her cabin. 'My doctor back home is going to be amazed,' she said."

Try BreathPlay techniques yourself. The next time you go out for a sustained walk, a bike ride, or a run, or perform any activity that requires any steady, rhythmic breathing, begin to experiment with different breathing patterns. As the name says, play with your breathing and learn to manipulate it. Try three stages on your outbreath and two on your inbreath, or try five on the outbreath and two on the inbreath. The secret is to find a breath pattern that you are comfortable with, keeping it an odd number of stages.

Enough people have spoken favorably of BreathPlay to make it worth investigating. Many of the exercises are fun and easy to do, and the results may surprise you. If what's being proposed is done so in a safe and responsible manner—and BreathPlay certainly is—then give it a try. There's nothing to lose, but a whole lot you might gain.

KEEPING TRACK OF GAINS

Within a few days you should see and feel the positive benefits of breathing exercises. However, with a peak-flow meter you can instantly and accurately gauge your daily progress. The meters are inexpensive and easy to use and record your peak expiratory flow. In addition to helping you chart your performance, a drop in your peak-flow meter reading will make you aware of the need for medication well in advance of acute asthma. See chapter 8 for more information on peak-flow meters.

RELAXATION

Dr. Leo Leonidas also emphasizes with his patients the importance of trying to remain relaxed at the onset of an asthma episode. He has developed a number of useful techniques that help reduce stress while promoting a calming effect. "Many children and some adults panic when they have asthma," he says, "which makes the situation worse. One of the basic problems during asthma is that the smooth muscles around the bronchial tubes go into spasm. Panic and stress then make the spasm even greater.

"When you get excited, nervous, or stressed, you start breathing fast and shallow—you don't move much air in and out of your lungs. This is hyperventilation. Your chest muscles get tight, and your diaphragm can't work right. You need to start some relaxation techniques in order to alleviate the hyperventilation."

Dr. Leonidas is a strong believer in using breathing techniques to help reduce the panic of asthma; he doesn't think that enough physicians emphasize their importance. Relaxation and stress-reduction methods are also ways of preventing asthma. "A relaxed body and mind can help in two ways," he says. "They can lessen the spasm of the smooth muscles and also reduce the oxygen requirement of the body. When you feel stressed or your early asthma symptoms are coming, begin relaxation techniques along with your asthma medications."

Air Wise, a publication of the National Institutes of Health, gives an effective relaxation method that Dr. Leonidas recommends you practice at least twice a day or as often as you need it when you're not having any asthma symptoms:

Lie on your back and concentrate on your feet. Feel the bones inside your feet. Feel the muscles that move these bones. Tense your feet by curling your toes. Now relax your toes. Feel a soothing, tingling sensation that comes into your feet. Notice the difference between when your feet were tense and the way they are after the exercise.

Now tense your legs. Point your toes and lift your legs off the floor an inch or two. Now let your legs drop. Let all the tightness drop out.

Now tighten your fists. Clench them really hard. Now let them go limp.

Now imagine that you're a turtle. Shrug your shoulders up toward your head into your shell. Feel the tension around your neck. Count to five and let all the tension go away.

Just lie there and imagine that you're in a warm bathtub.

Move your jaw back and forth, then let your jaw and tongue go limp.

Very gently check your whole body with your mind. Find any part of your body that's not fully relaxed. Take a deep breath, and when you let the air go out, imagine that you're blowing the air right out through your skin where there's any tension or tightness.

Start at the top of your head. See if there's a place where tension is still hiding out. Move down your shoulders, your arms, and your chest.

Keep breathing slowly and quietly.

Try to imagine that you feel very warm and comfortable. Just try to let your breath flow in and out without any problem.

AEROBIC WORKOUTS

While his team continues to run through plays on the field, Danny Boniface, a thirteen-year-old Fair Lawn, New Jersey, football player, jogs over to the sidelines and uses his inhaler. This medication is just one of several that Danny has been taking daily since he was two years old to help control his severe asthma. After looking at Danny's roomful of MVP football and baseball trophies (Danny is also captain and all-star catcher of his local baseball team), it's difficult to believe that this boy has spent almost as much of his life in doctors' offices and hospitals as he has on the playing fields. "He's really something," says Lori Boniface, Danny's mother, who started Danny in Pee Wee football in the first grade even though his asthma was so bothersome. "One time Danny was in the emergency room after a really severe attack and I thought that he'd never make it out. He was there for seventy-two hours."

When Danny was first diagnosed as having asthma, Lori Boniface thought that asthma was something that would go away, like the measles or chicken pox. She soon learned differently as Danny's health seemed to fluctuate with the seasons. She and her husband began to read all they could about asthma and talked about it to everyone, from doctors to other parents of children with asthma.

When it came to running around outside with other neighborhood children, playing tag, baseball, and football, Danny's parents felt exercise and sports would help their son become less introverted—they felt that the asthma was making him extremely shy—as well as possibly help his overall condition.

"If Danny was allowed to just sit around and watch TV or use computer games, I'm sure that he would be much worse off now," says Mrs. Boniface. "By being so involved in sports, he's doing something that he enjoys, he's participating with a team going through rigorous workouts, and he's growing physically and socially. We couldn't be happier with his progress."

Overall, the Bonifaces feel that sports have helped their son by making him stronger, but also by enabling him to better handle what asthma does to him. "Just because Danny has bad asthma doesn't mean that he should have to stay by the sidelines," says Mrs. Boniface. "With regular medication and monitoring, there's no reason why he can't participate. If he gets in trouble, he just cuts back a bit."

Danny often has to miss school and league games because of his asthma. Still, Mrs. Boniface can't see the virtue in sheltering a child with asthma who wants so much to play sports. "If sports is something a child enjoys doing, if he's gifted at it, then he has to do it," she says. "You should never treat a child with asthma like an invalid, because they aren't. Sports will help build confidence and boost self-esteem. If you hold a child back because of your own fears, then you're performing a great disservice to the child."

There are approximately three million children in the United States with asthma. Like Danny Boniface, even those who have severe asthma should be encouraged to begin exercising. Thanks to a better understanding of asthma and improved medications, this exercise can even include distance running, an activity often considered off-limits by many physicians. "We were apprehensive at first when it came to sports," says Mrs. Boniface, "but Danny joined right in and has exceeded all our wildest dreams. He doesn't feel sorry for himself because he has asthma. He understands that asthma is his problem and he's learned to manage it."

Parents of children with asthma as well as adults with asthma are often apprehensive about starting an exercise program or participating in sports because they're afraid the asthma will get worse. "One can overcome the fear of exercising by joining an organized exercise program that's led by someone who is both skilled and sensitive to the problems of patients with asthma," explains Henry Milgrom, M.D., associate professor of pediatrics at the University of Colorado and a staff physician at the National Jewish Center for Immunology and Respiratory Medicine in Denver. "By getting over these fears and apprehensions, children with asthma can begin to forget about their asthma and self-imposed limitations and start to have fun with their peers."

The key word in any exercise or sports program has to be fun, explains Dr. Milgrom, who works on a daily basis with children with severe asthma. "The main thing about exercise is not to prepare someone for competitive athletics. Exercise doesn't necessarily mean doing calisthenics or endurance running, either. Exercise for someone with asthma can consist of going outside, running around, and having fun. There's nothing wrong if some children don't like organized sports. In that case, they'll usually respond well if their parents accompany them regularly on outings to fly a kite, throw a ball around, or go for a walk."

HOW TO START AN
EXERCISE PROGRAM

In creating an exercise routine that you'll be able to maintain throughout the year, you must follow certain basic principles. These include:

1. See your doctor for a medical evaluation.
2. Make fitness a regular, year-round activity.
3. Set realistic goals for yourself.
4. Select your activities carefully.
5. Don't skip warm-ups and cool-downs.

6. Don't be compulsive about your exercise program.

7. Add variety to your workouts.

See Your Doctor

Before beginning an exercise program, check with your asthma physician. If your case is already well documented, a medical evaluation prior to exercise may consist of a conversation covering goals and premedication. If your physician has some doubts about your capabilities, he or she may want you to take an exercise tolerance test in order to evaluate your lung function and capacity.

If your physician knows how to treat your condition but doesn't know how to help you lead a healthier life through exercise, start your search for a new doctor (see chapter 8). Ideally, this doctor should be a regular exerciser, or should have experience working with athletes who have asthma. Finding the right doctor may take time and effort, but it will be worth it. Your physician will give you advice and monitor your progress. If some difficulties arise, it's your physician who can best help you by changing your medication or by slightly altering or completely modifying your exercise program to suit your capabilities.

Make Fitness a Regular, Year-Round Activity

Physical fitness can be achieved and maintained if your exercise is rhythmic, continuous, and vigorous. In order for exercise to have any sustained benefit, you must exercise for at least twenty minutes three times a week. Working out once a week has not been found to have any sustained fitness benefits and can also lead to injury because of the demands made on the unconditioned body.

If you really want to start having fun and participate in sports or exercise, don't let "time" stand in your way. If you gave only thirty minutes per session, three times a week, it would take one and a half hours out of a total 168 possible hours in the week. It's really not hard to get in the time. In addition to running, swimming, or taking aerobic dance classes, I do 200 sit-ups a day. It takes about one second to do each one and I'm all finished in just three minutes. Review your schedule and see where you can fit in exercise with the least amount of distraction. Try walking to work or squeezing in a run during your lunch break or after work. If you drive a car, park it several blocks from your destination and walk. Ride an exercise bike at home while watching TV. The opportunities are endless.

Because of work or travel obligations, there are many times when I can't get to my favorite park for a run or make it to the pool, but I still get in my workouts. Instead of taking the elevator, I'll walk up the stairs to my apartment. If I know that my day will be filled with appointments, I'll get up earlier in the morning and exercise, taking care of it right away instead of hoping that I'll be able to exercise at my customary time later in the day. When I'm on the road, I always take along my running shoes, and I make sure that the hotel I stay in has a good exercise room or, even better, a swimming pool.

Set Realistic Goals for Yourself

If you're out of shape (i.e., you wheeze after going up a flight of stairs or you can't walk a half mile without reaching for your inhaler), then you have the most to gain from an exercise program. Don't be discouraged after your first workout if your ribs are sore and your leg muscles feel like rubber: Your body can't be changed instantly. Don't be hard on yourself; be willing to accept setbacks and disappointments without hanging up your sweats for good. Only after being on an exercise routine for at least two months can you step back and objectively assess your progress and changes. After the Olympics, I took up running, and it took me a year and a half of regular workouts, gradually increasing my pace and distance, to reach the point where I now feel comfortable and satisfied with my running. And I had just finished competing in the Olympics!

It is a big disadvantage to work out by yourself because you have to be your own coach, inspiration, and motivating force. So take the time to sit down and write out the short-term and long-term goals you would like to achieve from your exercise program. Short-term goals should bolster your spirits, motivate you, and encourage you to go back day after day to your exercise program. These goals should be attainable in one to twelve months and might, for example, include some of the following:

- Being able to walk/jog one and a half miles without stopping; twenty minutes for the distance is a good goal
- Gaining more stamina and energy in your daily life
- Carrying bags of groceries into the house without getting winded
- Losing ten pounds of body weight in ten weeks
- Swimming three miles in a week

Your long-term goals should be exciting and challenging—and attainable in one year to eighteen months. Some examples of long-term goals include:

- Fully integrating your exercise program into your life so that it becomes "automatic"
- Dropping one minute off your best mile running time
- Pedaling 5,000 miles on your bike in one year
- Achieving your "ideal" weight
- Exercising continuously for twenty minutes without bringing on an asthma episode

Goal setting is important in continuing your exercise program. Once you are able to define what you really want from your fitness program, you will be better able to achieve your aims. Also, when setting goals, don't neglect the psychological benefits of exercise. Researchers believe that most people exercise not so much because they're worried about their heart or overall health, but because they're concerned about trying to realize their full potential. Therefore, any program that you design needs to be part aerobic to strengthen your heart and lungs, but it also has to be challenging so that you can adequately test yourself. It's a delicate balance to achieve. If your exercise program doesn't help you achieve your psychological goals, or if it turns out to be too challenging, you'll end up quitting your program in no time.

After you've consulted with your physician and have written down your goals, put some reins on your enthusiasm. All exercise programs have to be started *gradually* and with caution. Fitness takes time and can't be achieved in a week or two. As Dr. Jim Angel, the chairman of the Department of Health and Physical Education at Samford University, points out, "It took you years to get out of condition, so don't expect to get it all back in a few weeks. It's a slow process."

Be patient. Be diligent in your approach to exercise. However, by exercising at least three times a week for at least twenty uninterrupted minutes at a stretch, you'll absolutely start to see changes in how you feel physically and emotionally.

Select Your Activities Carefully

It's important for both children and adults to understand that there are some activities that are less likely to trigger asthma than others. Swimming, which is an excellent aerobic activity that will greatly increase lung capacity, is also the activity least likely to cause asthma because of the moist, humid air found in a pool or open water. Swimming includes water polo, synchronized swimming, and diving. Activities such as walking, wrestling, sprinting, baseball, badminton, doubles tennis, and other sports that are stop-and-go by nature are also recommended because they produce little bronchoconstriction.

When selecting appropriate activities consider the levels of dust, air pollution, and pollen levels where the activity is going to be carried out. It's good to have a fallback activity you can execute in an air-conditioned environment when outdoor conditions prove unacceptable.

But the most important factor in choosing a sport is to find one you love. You'll get more satisfaction from it and will stick with it in the long run. Even though the activity or sport that you choose may trigger asthma (such as distance running or basketball), remember that many athletes with asthma have succeeded in these sports by working with their physician and learning how to manage their asthma with medication.

Don't Skip Warm-ups and Cool-downs

A warm-up is a period of slow, easy exercise that will gradually raise your body temperature, gently stretch your muscles and prepare them for exercise, accelerate your heart rate, and increase blood flow to the muscles. You're ready to begin your workout session when you are perspiring lightly or when your heart rate has accelerated twenty to thirty beats above the resting rate.

Workouts should always start with a warm-up period of no less than five to ten minutes, sometimes even longer if you find that you need it. Stretching exercises should be included to prepare your joints for upcoming demands. Many athletes with asthma have found that a good warm-up lessens the impact of EIB, often eliminating wheezing or chest tightness. Good warm-ups include full breathing exercises, calisthenics, slow jogging, slow walking, skipping rope, and easy laps in the pool. You can also do your sport at a greatly reduced intensity as a warm-up. For example, walk through the first five minutes of a basketball game to get ready to play hard, or walk the first half-mile of a planned run.

Cooling down properly after your workout is just as important as a good warm-up. Your aim is to slowly return your cardiovascular system to almost a preworkout condition. Don't come to a complete stop after a vigorous workout, because it will cause a quick drop in blood pressure, which can put a strain on the heart and also bring on a potential oxygen shortage to the brain. In extreme cases, dizziness or fainting can result. By cooling down, decreasing the intensity of your workout for five or ten minutes before you actually stop exercising, you will decrease the likelihood of a drop in blood pressure.

Cooling down seems an unnecessary ritual, even to some top athletes, and many foolishly choose to skip it. However, the effects will sometimes show up in their next workout. They feel stiff, their muscles ache, and their workouts are not what they could be.

Muscle soreness and poor results discourage many who are trying to make sports and fitness a part of their lives. Skipping the cool-down can undermine the firmest resolve, so don't neglect it!

Don't Be Compulsive About Your Exercise Program

If your exercise program is to succeed, you have to learn at which intensity level to begin and how much to push yourself. Many people, especially the newcomers to exercise, make the mistake of working out at too high an intensity, thinking that the harder they strain and the greater the muscle pain they feel, the more beneficial their workout will be. This can be a big mistake, one that can eventually lead them to quit.

Exercise shouldn't be looked at as hard work. For activities such as swimming, walking, running, cycling, or skating to be beneficial, they should be performed in a *rhythmical, vigorous, and continuous manner*. If you only concentrate on the vigorous aspect of exercise, pushing yourself hard all of the time, you'll become frustrated and disillusioned when you can't achieve your exercise goals, and eventually will push yourself right out of exercise.

Elite athletes can be just as guilty of overstressing their bodies when they cross the delicate boundary that separates exercise from overexercise. They suddenly find that they are more susceptible to muscle pulls, they develop colds that seem to linger, and their workouts become an ordeal. Tracy Sundlund, the top track-and-field coach who's prepared numerous athletes for the Olympics, runs across this all the time in the course of his work. "I find in working with elite athletes," says Sundlund, "that even though they might be at their best stage competitively, they're not necessarily as healthy as they could be. This is because they're so close to the edge. It's like walking blindfolded alongside a cliff. If you're a half-inch from the edge and you take that extra step, you're over the side with no coming back."

To compound the problem, these athletes often try to exercise through an injury they may have developed because of the intensity of their training. Unfortunately, what they're working toward isn't better health but a seat on the sidelines and a sure visit to the doctor.

When you want to exercise a bit more strenuously than before, a good rule of thumb is to increase the time you spend exercising, the distance you walk, or the amount of weight you lift by no more than 10 percent over your previous level. Anything above 10 percent will take you from a safe situation to a stressful one your body won't be prepared for, with an injury often the end result.

Add Variety to Your Workouts

By challenging yourself to an array of physical tasks during the week, your interest in exercise will remain high and you'll eagerly look forward to each workout. Give circuit training a try. This is a system of exercise using different machines or activities during the same workout. Riding a bike for ten minutes, running for another ten, and then swimming for ten more minutes are an example of circuit exercise. Circuits can also be made using various weight machines or stationary exercise equipment.

A NOTE ABOUT THE EXERCISE PROGRAMS

The success of your exercise program depends on you. You have to learn to listen to your body, learn how you feel during and after a workout, both physically and mentally, and understand what makes you feel that way. Pay attention to your overall condition— signs of early fatigue or how sore you are.

You should never be bullied into completing a preplanned exercise routine that you may have set up but don't feel prepared for. What's crucial to your success as a regular exerciser is that you're able to learn and then understand your body's reaction to a particular workout. For some, this understanding may come in a few weeks, but for most people, basic comprehension comes within a few months.

CHOOSING YOUR EXERCISE

Aerobic exercise is any type of continuous activity that involves the large muscle groups such as the legs and arms and thereby increases the needs of your heart and lungs for more oxygen. Researchers have documented that aerobic activities such as walking, running, swimming, bicycling, and aerobic dancing bring the most benefit to the cardiorespiratory system, improving overall fitness in the process.

The best exercise for you is one that you will stick with and enjoy. For many, convenience is also a factor. If you live near a health club that happens to have a swimming pool, then consider joining and starting a swimming program. If you live near a park, then walking or running might be for you. If you like the feeling of speed, bicycling could be a good exercise option.

In choosing your sport, you also have to consider your physical condition. See your doctor before beginning any exercise program. If you haven't exercised for a long time because of your asthma, swimming would be a good choice for a starter activity because the water and humid surroundings of the pool or seaside are excellent for people with asthma. Also, your body will be better protected from the jarring shocks of land-based impact activities. The chapters that follow this one provide you with a detailed look at the benefits of several different aerobic activities, as well as the equipment needed for basic workouts. Read closely, then try a sport, or several sports, that appeal to you. As your fitness level improves, you may want to consider cross training, concentrating, for example, on only one activity during the week but including several aerobic sports in your weekend workouts.

MOTIVATION TO EXERCISE AND STAY WITH IT

When it comes time to exercise, do you frequently find yourself putting it off? According to Art Turock, a Seattle-based motivational expert, the only legitimate excuses for not exercising three times a week all year round are severe illness, injury, or a difficult pregnancy. Any other excuses, no matter how valid they might seem, just don't count.

"What gets in the way and keeps most people from exercising is their amazing ability to create for themselves perceptions of difficulty," says Turock. "And as long as this perceived difficulty continues to exceed the perceived value of exercise, then exercise will always be inconsistent at best." Once a person comes to place a high value on fitness, there aren't any difficulties that can't be overcome.

Turock believes that there are two groups of exercisers: those who are "committed" and those who are merely "interested" in exercising. Too frequently, the interested exercisers carry on internal monologues about whether or not optimum conditions exist for exercise at that particular time. By creating mental traps—excuses such as cold or hot weather, or that they're too tired or have too much work to do—these exercisers prevent themselves from achieving or sustaining their target fitness levels. Does this sound like you?

"Whenever you come up with excuses not to exercise, you're actually trying to do what's easiest for you," says Turock. "Exercise often isn't easy, but committed exercisers will exercise no matter what difficulty is presented because they know what they're getting from exercise far exceeds everything else. The so-called difficulties that may sidetrack them are really insignificant in comparison.

"The bottom line is that when people are committed, they're all-powerful. When they're only interested in exercising, they may follow through, but only if circumstances permit. With this attitude, it's easy to see why this group doesn't get results."

Committed exercisers look for ways to fit sports activities into their day, not reasons to cancel. For example, a runner will find a treadmill to use indoors during the pollen season when his or her peak-flow-meter reading is down 15 percent despite increased medication. Don't let excuses rule you, says Turock. Willpower is something that everyone possesses and that's what it takes to exercise.

Family obligations, your job, or your asthma should not keep you from your weekly exercise appointments. The issue here is not about having enough time in the day or being worried about your asthma, says Turock. "It really comes down to being committed to your exercise program. If you're committed to taking care of your health, then you'll find the time to exercise."

If you have a spouse who doesn't understand why you're exercising and complains about your absences from home, or if you have a parent or close friend who questions why you exercise even though you have severe asthma, it's time to sit down and clear the air. "I call my own exercise time a period of rejuvenation, a second wind, a physical and mental recharging," says Turock. "If you can explain that you're able to give more to your family because exercise relieves you of built-up stress from the job, that you now have more energy, are in better health, and are in good spirits because of it, I think you'll get your point across." Over time your family member or friend will see the results.

Similarly, you need to explain to a worried parent that even though you might experience some wheezing during exercise or a game, this is no cause for alarm. Tell them that you are able to handle these flare-ups, that you have worked out procedures with your doctor, and that with a little medication you can soon be back exercising with no ill effects. Communication with people close to you can help in getting them to support your commitment to fitness rather than pull you away from it.

A good way to ensure your success as a regular exerciser is to assign someone to be your fitness coach. Turock, a former ninety-seven-pound weakling who was transformed physically and mentally through weight lifting and long-distance running, believes that having a "coach," a person who understands your weekly exercise goals and is tough-minded enough not to let you make excuses for not achieving them, will help add consistency to your sessions.

"This coach doesn't have to work out with you," explains Turock, "but should check in twice a week to see how you're doing. Your coach can keep you committed when you're having a bad day and all the excuses are looking real. He or she shouldn't put up with your excuses for missing workouts. Instead, your coach should point out how flimsy your excuses are and help you reschedule sessions."

HOME WORKOUTS:
THE NO-FRILLS APPROACH

A regular exercise program doesn't have to be a complicated affair that involves joining a health club or spa. There are many simple, easy-to-do routines that can help improve your aerobic capacity with a minimum of expense and time. Best of all, these workouts can be done at home with equipment as basic as exercise clothing and a mat for calisthenics and stretching. For those who want to invest a little money, a quality exercise bike, rowing machine, cross-country ski simulator, stair-climbing machine, or motorized treadmill will do a lot to enhance your fitness.

If you're serious about your health and fitness, purchasing one or more pieces of exercise equipment makes sense. With the advent of reliable, affordable, and compact home exercise equipment, you can exercise in the privacy of your bedroom, cellar, or garage, or wherever you have the available space. No longer do you have to be at the mercy of pollen, humidity, or cold weather. Of course, these home machines can't do the exercise for you, but they do offer the means to safely and efficiently achieve aerobic conditioning, strength, and flexibility—whenever you want to exercise.

The following are two basic exercise circuits that you can set up in your home workout area that will maximize your exercise time and help you to achieve substantial fitness improvements. Repetitions and workout times given are only suggestions. If the workouts prove too strenuous, scale them down to your current fitness level, gradually increasing your time and intensity over a period of weeks.

EXERCISE CIRCUIT WITHOUT EQUIPMENT

Needed: Workout clothing, exercise mat.

1. **Warm-up:** Jog in place for 2 minutes, or do jumping jacks for 2 minutes, to elevate heart rate and increase core body temperature.

2. **Flexibility:** Roll out the exercise mat and stretch for 5 minutes, working key body parts from head to toe. An excellent sourcebook is *Stretching* by Bob Anderson ($9.95 plus $3 shipping; to order, call 1-800-333-1307, or write Stretching Inc., PO Box 767, Palmer Lake, CO 80133).

A Basic Everyday Stretching Routine

Use the following everyday stretches to fine-tune your muscles. This is a general routine that emphasizes stretching and relaxing the muscles most frequently used during the normal day-to-day activities. It is taken from *Stretching* by Bob Anderson, illustrated by Jean Anderson, copyright © 1980, Shelter Publications.

A. *Lying groin stretch*: Relax, with knees bent and the soles of your feet together. This comfortable position will stretch your groin. Hold for 30 seconds. Let the pull of gravity do the stretching.

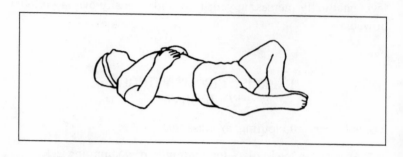

B. *Lower back flattener*: To relieve tension in the lower back area, tighten your butt (gluteus) muscles and, at the same time, tighten your abdominal muscles to flatten your lower back. Hold the tension for 5 to 8 seconds, then relax. Repeat 2 to 3 times. Concentrate on maintaining constant muscle contraction. This pelvic tilting exercise will strengthen the butt and abdominal muscles so that you are able to sit and stand with good posture.

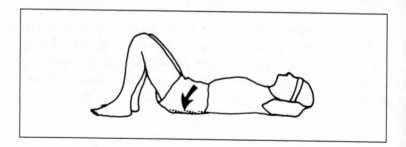

C. *Upper spine stretch*: Interlace your fingers behind your head at about ear level. Now, use the power of your arms to slowly pull your head forward until you feel a slight stretch in the back of your neck. Hold for 5 to 10 seconds, then slowly return to the original starting position. Do this 3 to 4 times to gradually loosen the upper spine and neck.

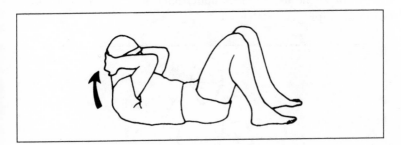

D. *Elongation stretch:* Extend your arms overhead and straighten out your legs. Now reach as far as is comfortable in opposite directions with your arms and legs. Stretch for 5 seconds, then relax.

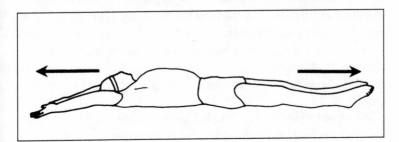

E. *Groin stretch:* Put the soles of your feet together and hold on to your toes. Gently pull yourself forward, bending from the hips, until you feel a good stretch in your groin. Hold for 40 seconds. Do not make the stretch movement from head and shoulders; move from the hips.

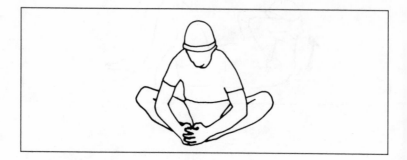

F. *Spinal twist:* This is good for the upper back, lower back, side of hips, and rib cage. Sit with your left leg straight. Bend your right leg, cross your right foot over and rest it to the outside of your left knee. Then bend your left elbow and rest it on the outside of your upper right thigh, just above the knee. During the stretch, use the elbow to keep this leg stationary with controlled pressure to the inside.

With your right hand resting behind you, slowly turn your head to look over your right shoulder and at the same time rotate your upper body toward your right hand and arm. As you turn your upper body, think of turning your hips in the same direction (though your hips won't move because your left elbow is keeping this right leg stationary). Hold for 15 seconds. Do for both sides.

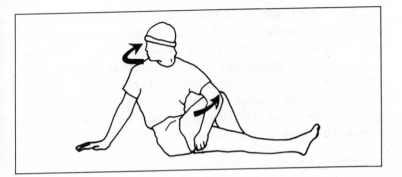

G. *Hamstring stretch:* Straighten your left leg with the sole of your right foot slightly touching the inside of the left thigh. Slowly bend forward from the hips toward the foot of the straight leg until you create the slightest feeling of a stretch. Hold your foot for 20 seconds. After the stretch feeling has diminished, bend a bit more forward from the hips. Hold this developmental stretch for 25 seconds. Switch sides and stretch the right leg in the same manner.

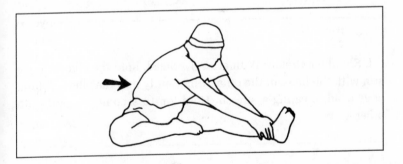

H. *Calf stretch:* Stand a little back from a solid support and lean on it with your forearms, head resting on hands. Bend one leg and place your foot on the ground in front of you, with the other leg straight behind. Slowly move your hips forward, keeping your lower back flat. Be sure to keep the heel of the straight leg on the ground, with toes pointed straight ahead or slightly turned in as you hold the stretch. Hold an easy stretch for 30 seconds, then stretch the other leg.

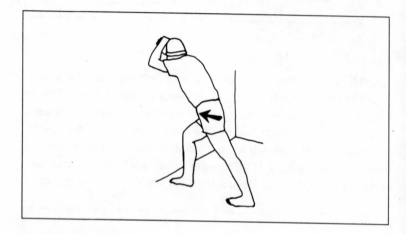

I. *Shoulder stretch:* With arms overhead, hold the elbow of one arm with the hand of the other arm. Gently pull the elbow behind your head, creating a stretch. Hold for 15 seconds. Repeat with other arm.

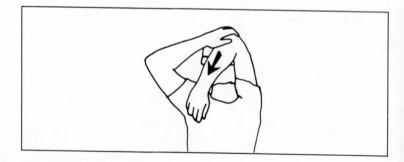

3. **Aerobic:** Jog in place or skip rope for 5 minutes.

4. **Strength:** Get on your mat and do either 20 sit-ups with knees bent, feet on floor, or 20 push-ups. If this is difficult, lower the number of repetitions, but begin to increase them by one repetition a week in ensuing weeks.

5. **Aerobic:** Jog in place or skip rope for 5 minutes.

6. **Strength:** If you previously did sit-ups, do 20 push-ups this time.

7. **Aerobic:** Jog in place or skip rope for 5 minutes.

8. **Strength:** Do 10 sit-ups or push-ups.

9. **Aerobic:** Jog in place or skip rope for 5 minutes, going much slower in the final 2 minutes as a cool-down phase to redirect blood flow to the heart and help the muscles to recover.

10. **Flexibility:** Stretch major body parts for 5 to 10 minutes to increase muscle length and flexibility.

WORKOUT CIRCUIT WITH EQUIPMENT

Needed: Workout clothing, exercise mat, home gym equipment.

1. **Warm-up:** Go at a slow pace for 2 minutes on your home exercise equipment (bike, rower, treadmill, cross-country ski simulator, stair climber) to raise your core body temperature.

2. **Flexibility:** Stretch for 5 minutes, paying attention to body parts that will be principally exercised on your machine.

3. **Aerobic:** Exercise nonstop for 20 minutes on your exercise equipment. Keep your pace steady, with resistance set at a level that doesn't leave you gasping or straining.

If you have another piece of aerobic equipment, try switching to this piece after 10 minutes. This will let you work different body parts and add interest to the workout by providing a new challenge.

In the final 2 minutes of the workout, cool down by reducing your pace and speed to redirect blood flow back to the heart and help the muscles to recover.

5. **Flexibility:** Stretch major body parts for 5 to 10 minutes to increase muscle length and flexibility.

HOME GYM WORKOUT TIPS

You'll often have days when your workouts seem to be dragging and you can't gather much enthusiasm. One of the biggest obstacles to a home exercise program is boredom. A good trick to help add some zest to your workouts is to listen to music, watch television, or read a magazine or book as you exercise. The time seems to pass more quickly and more pleasantly when your mind is otherwise occupied. You'll also find that you won't be constantly looking at your watch, counting down the minutes until the workout is over.

SWIMMING

Swimming, as I have pointed out before, is one of the best exercises for people with asthma because of the warm, humid environment presented by the water. In addition, swimming forces you to develop your breathing muscles, as you inhale deeply and quickly when your head breaks the surface of the water and then exhale completely underwater.

Not only do the rhythmic movements of swimming gently work the body's major muscle groups—arms, legs, and trunk—but swimming also helps develop the heart and lungs. Because of this, swimming is a great activity for those already in good physical condition and a fine exercise for those at the lowest rung of the fitness ladder.

Jill Abrams first began swimming in her hometown of Eagle Creek, Alaska, when she was six years old. Over the next twelve years, Abrams went on to set eighteen state age-group records in the freestyle and butterfly while leading her high-school team to forty-eight straight dual-meet victories and three state championships.

One day during her junior year in high school, Jill lifted weights before swim practice and then went out for a run. She remembers that the air was particularly cold and dry that afternoon. Later, the swim workout wasn't going well for her, and after a few laps it felt as if her throat was contracting, getting smaller and smaller. It suddenly became more difficult to breathe. "I had to get out of the pool. I was so scared," she recalls. "I didn't know what was happening to me."

That night her family physician examined her. EIB was diagnosed and medication prescribed. "I wasn't going to let asthma control my life," says the determined Abrams. "I wanted to win a college scholarship and nothing was going to stop me."

Jill brought her inhaler with her to practice every day, taking several puffs twenty minutes before getting in the pool and then leaving the inhaler on the pool deck just in case she needed it again. "The medication usually prevents my asthma," she says, "but it doesn't always work. I don't really know why."

One time Jill found that she couldn't get in enough air in the middle of a backstroke competition. "I just forced myself to relax and not panic. I was able to finish the race and came in second, four seconds off my best time."

This is typical of the way Jill Abrams has managed her asthma. She's always on top of it and doesn't let it control her life. After leading her team to yet another state championship in her senior year, Jill capped off the year by winning a prestigious Presidential Scholar award, and in addition was selected as the 1987 Asthma Athlete of the Year. This national scholarship award presented by The Asthma and Allergy Foundation of America is given each year to the top male and female high-school athlete who, in spite of asthma, reaches a high level of achievement both in the classroom and on the playing field. "Asthma can be a big roadblock, but it shouldn't stop you," says Jill, who now competes for the University of Maine swim team.

Although swimming won't make asthma disappear, as Jill Abrams found out, it's an excellent activity for someone with asthma because it works the upper body so well. Contrary to popular belief, in freestyle (crawl) swimming most of the forward propulsion comes from the arms and shoulders, with the legs and feet used only sparingly to keep the body horizontal in the water and to save oxygen. A regular swim program builds up the breathing muscles, increasing aerobic capacity in the process.

There are many advantages to a year-round swimming program for someone with asthma. Since the body is immersed in water that's much cooler than the body core temperature, a hard workout won't bring on the overheating of land-based activities such as running and cycling. Also, during the scorching days of summer when elevated pollution and pollen levels might be high enough to trigger asthma in someone who attempts to work out, swimmers don't seem to be bothered.

THE POOL

For many of you, workouts and competitions will be done in swimming pools that have a water temperature of about 80 degrees F. Olympic-sized pools, also called long-course pools, are 50 meters long and have lane markers and gutters to cut down on the wave action of the water. Pools that are 25 yards long are called short-course pools and are generally identical to the longer pools except that you have to swim twice as many laps as you do in the 50-meter pools to cover the same distance. Pools shorter than 15 yards are generally unacceptable for swim workouts because you'll be spending most of your time turning at the end walls.

Most pools have painted lines on the bottom. Follow these lines as you swim and you'll stay on a straight course. More than one person can easily swim in a lane; when I worked out with my swim team, we would have up to fifty people swimming in the 25-yard pool at one time. To pass, you pull out just as you would if you were in a car and you try to get by quickly. If you are the one going slowly, you let the faster swimmers pass you at the turnaround point. Three swimmers should be able to pass each other through the lane without too much trouble.

OPEN WATER

Open-water swimming is not like swimming in a pool. There are no lines or lane markers and no walls to hold on to when you need to catch your breath. The first time out of the pool and in open water can present some anxious moments, but if you keep your wits about you and relax, there should be no problems.

A good recommendation is to wear a bathing cap that is highly visible from a distance. Not only will the bathing cap keep in your body heat and help you stay warm, but it will also signal boaters that a swimmer is in the area.

Pacing is important if you are to enjoy your swim. Start out slowly so you'll have enough energy at the finish. And be sure to swim with a friend. You'll enjoy the company, and if you should happen to experience any difficulty during your workout, there will be someone immediately at your side to help you.

SUGGESTED SWIM WORKOUTS

Going to the pool and just swimming lap after lap can become boring. (See pages 181–185 for pool exercise geared to those who aren't strong lap swimmers.) By having a set workout in mind before you start, however, you can make your pool workouts more interesting and efficient.

If you don't belong to an organized swim team or program, make up your own workouts. Your first goal should be to swim three to four times a week, establishing a swimming base through long steady distance (LSD) training by trying to cover at least 40 meters in a minute. If this pace is too demanding, don't give up. With practice you can achieve it.

Stroke choice is yours. While most will opt for the crawl (free-style) because it's the most efficient stroke, try sidestroke or breast-stroke if either is to your liking. Start out slowly, going one lap at a time in the pool and fully resting before starting out again. Aim for swimming 100 meters, or four laps, in the pool doing the crawl and then call it a day. If the crawl is too tiring, switch to the breaststroke or sidestroke.

If you feel asthma coming on, don't be embarrassed to stop and rest for a while. Use your inhaler if needed. If you're simply tired, then get out of the pool and walk slowly to the other end, get in, and start swimming again.

You may have setbacks along the way in your swimming program. If you do develop asthma and miss a few workouts, don't try to pick up exactly where you left off. Instead, take it slow. Aim for about half the number of laps you swam before your episode and then start building up from there.

Betty DeMont, the mother of Rick DeMont, recalls many times when her son had to be scratched from swim meets and sent home because of his asthma. Her son was upset, of course, but he never looked back. "It was disappointing for him not to be able to race," she says, "but I didn't pamper him. There were other swim meets, and he would do his best and try to be ready for them."

As your swimming ability increases along with your strength and endurance, you will need to use little tricks to keep workouts interesting and fresh. For example, make the highlight of your last workout the goal of your next workout. This could mean swimming as many laps as you did the last time, then trying to tack on a few more. Or keep up your previous lap pace, then try to lower it slightly.

If you're a beginning swimmer, an easy goal might be trying to do two laps continuously before resting. Decrease your rest time as you feel yourself getting more fit. After a month or so, your goal can be to try to do four continuous laps.

Suggested Swim Schedule

Week	Distance	Workout
1–2	100 yards	Four 25-yard swims at your own pace, with a 15-second rest between 25s
3–8	200 yards	Two 100-yard swims at your own pace, with 25-to-30-second rests between 100s
9–16	800 yards	Four 200-yard swims at your own pace, with 25-to-30-second rests between 200s

WATER EXERCISES

The following exercises were designed to be done in the water. As you will see, many of them involve large sweeping movements. For maximum benefit, it's important that you perform them at your own pace and to the best of your ability. As you will discover, these exercises will help improve your cardiovascular fitness and increase your muscular strength and the range of motion in your joints.

The beauty of these water exercises is that you don't need a lap pool to perform them; any backyard pool will do just fine. Water exercises are ideal for anyone with a weight problem, since the water reduces the effects of gravity, making you feel "light" while exercising in the water. Also, exercising in the water provides passive resistance. While it's tougher to exercise and move through water than it is to perform a similar exercise in a gym, water is gentle. It doesn't jolt the tendons or joints, which makes water exercise ideal for someone with an injury who still wants to stay in shape while the injury heals, or someone who wants a hard workout without the pounding he or she would get on land.

1. Stand with your back to the wall. (a) Raise one leg up, knee bent. Extend leg out, stretching back of leg. Bring leg back to standing position. Repeat with opposite leg. (b) Stretch one leg straight out in front of you and raise it as high as you can. Sweep it out to the side, then pull it down toward the starting position. Repeat with other leg.

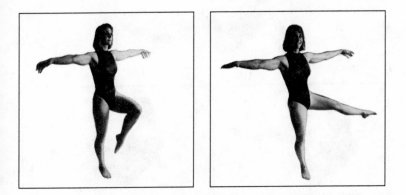

2. Stand next to the pool wall, holding the wall with one arm, the other extended for balance. Keeping your feet in the same place and your stomach pulled in, touch your hip to the wall. Come back to the standing start position and swing your hip away from the wall. Repeat.

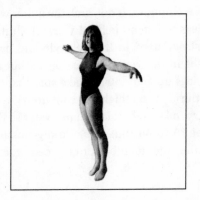

3. With your back against the wall, grab the gutter. (a) Let your legs float to the top. (b) Pull knees in toward chest. (c) From the hips, twist slowly to the left. Repeat on right side.

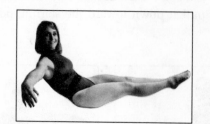

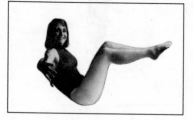 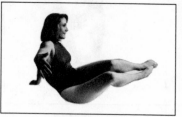

4. If you are in a lap pool and have a kickboard, you can do laps using these kick techniques. If not, grab the gutter with your hands, allowing your legs to extend behind you. (a) Flutter-kick. This is the basic kick stroke used in the freestyle and backstroke. Keep your legs straight in the water, knees locked but ankles relaxed, and move your legs up and down. Make sure that the kick motion originates from the hips and thighs and not from the knees. Stronger swimmers can try to keep their feet underwater so they don't make a splash. Repeat 20 to 40 times. (b) Do big-scissors kicks. Bring each leg out to the side, then back to the center, crossing slightly at the ankles.

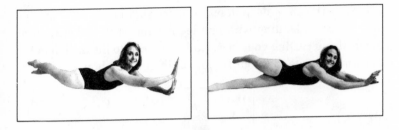

5. Face the wall and bring your knees up under your chest and put your feet on the wall. Using your feet, climb up the wall in several short steps. Walk back down the wall and repeat.

6. Grabbing the gutter, with legs extended behind you, use your arms to pull yourself toward the wall. Without letting go, push yourself away from the wall. Pull back and repeat.

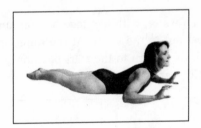

7. Standing chest-deep in water, place your hands on your hips and jump up, landing with one leg in front of the other. Repeat the drill, alternating your legs. Add your arms to the drill, moving the arm opposite the front leg forward with each hop.

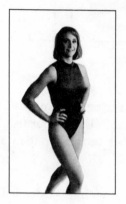

8. In chest-deep water, with feet together, (a) jump slightly, extending your feet out to the sides. At the same time, touch your palms overhead. (b) Return to the start position by bringing your hands to your sides and your legs together.

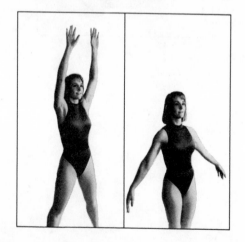

9. Standing in waist-deep water, (a) use your arms crawl-fashion to help pull you to the other side of the pool while walking. (b) Standing in slightly deeper water, walk back across the pool using your arms for balance and propulsion. (c) Walk backward while using your arms backstroke-style to help pull you to the other side of the pool. Note: To avoid unnecessary strain on your shoulders, rotate the shoulders 180 degrees with each stroke of freestyle and backstroke so that chest and back muscles are used.

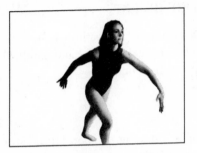 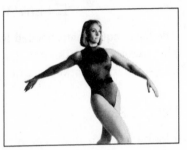

10. Lace your fingers behind your neck. Hop on one leg, bringing the other leg toward your chest while the opposite elbow touches the high knee. Walk forward as you alternate touching elbows and knees.

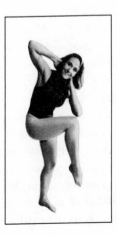

To cool down from these exercises, go to the shallow end of the pool and squat down, chest-deep in water, keeping your back as straight as possible. Pretend that you're a Russian dancer: Fold your arms over your chest and kick both legs out in front of you several times. Repeat the drill by kicking with just one leg at a time. Continue at least 5 minutes or until heart rate has returned to resting rate.

ESSENTIAL EQUIPMENT

The basic equipment needed for swimming is a bathing suit, goggles, and a cap. Training aids such as a kickboard or hand paddles can spice up a workout and improve technique.

Bathing Suit

I look for a suit that is comfortable yet snug. A good-fitting suit helps cut water drag and resistance and allows you to move through the water more efficiently. If you're going to be serious about your swimming, buy a racing suit made of nylon or Lycra. I prefer Lycra because the material stretches and doesn't cut or chafe the way nonstretch suits can. However, Lycra doesn't have the durability of nylon.

Goggles and Cap

To prevent red eyes—the sting and soreness of the eyes caused by pool chemicals and salt water—invest in a pair of swim goggles and wear them whenever you go into the water to work out. There are many swim-goggle models to choose from, but there is no "perfect" model or shape. Try on a pair in a sporting-goods store and make sure that they're comfortable and fit well. They should rest over the eye area, not fit so snugly that you're using a lot of suction to keep them on. If water falls in easily, try a different model.

If your goggles fog up in the water, either purchase a special defogging product available at most sporting-goods stores or use your own saliva to lightly coat the inside of the lenses.

A bathing cap keeps hair out of your eyes, protects your hair from the ravages of chlorinated water, and keeps your head warm in cool water. Washing your hair after each swim with a mild shampoo will clean your hair of sweat and of water that may have leaked in under your cap. You don't have to choose between long, healthy hair and swimming. I had hair past my shoulders for most of my fifteen years as a competitive swimmer. I never rinsed my hair in the pool; instead, I took my cap off when I was out of the pool and in the shower and made sure I conditioned my hair daily.

Optional Training Aids

KICKBOARD

A kickboard is a piece of buoyant Styrofoam that can be used in learning proper kicking motion or as a training device for improving leg strength. Many novice swimmers have difficulty swimming on their own for twenty continuous minutes; a kickboard helps them to stay afloat while concentrating on their kicking, enabling them to keep their heart rate up for the full time during the intense portion of their practice.

To use a kickboard, grip the front of the board and hold it out in front of you with your arms extended. All propulsion should come from your legs as you move through the water using a flutter kick (moving your legs up and down in a scissors motion).

HAND PADDLES

Hand paddles are rectangular sheets of plastic that you slip on your hands to give you more resistance as you swim, which strengthens the muscles of your back, arms, shoulders, and chest. These are really for more advanced swimmers who want to add strength to their swimming.

Using hand paddles will also teach you better stroke mechanics. If you attempt to cut your stroke short before the end of your pull phase in freestyle swimming, you will feel resistance as the slightly curved end of the paddle pulls back, separating the paddle from your hand.

WALKING AND RUNNING

WALKING

Walking, Hippocrates once said long ago, is man's best medicine, and recent medical research has confirmed his wisdom. The age-old tortoise of transportation, walking, is now gaining respect as the perfect exercise because it improves aerobic capacity, puts little stress on the tendons and muscles, can help control weight, and requires no special equipment or lessons. With fifty-five million Americans naming walking as their exercise of choice, it would seem that we're currently in the midst of a walking boom.

Walking, according to Dr. James Rippe, director of the exercise physiology laboratory at the University of Massachusetts Medical School, is the one physical activity that almost any person can take part in. This is as true for those who are seventy-five pounds over their recommended weight as it is for those who work out three times a week and compete in a variety of sports. "While walking is not the only thing that you can do for exercise, it is an effective way for most people to get exercise on a regular and continuing basis with little fear of injury."

According to Dr. Rippe, the increased awareness in health and exercise that was brought on by the running boom in the 1970s was beneficial for a certain segment of American society. "Unfortunately," says Rippe, "a fifty-five-year-old sedentary male with some degree of coronary artery disease can't relate to a marathoner or a triathlete."

Steve Jonas, M.D., a fifty-year-old professor of preventive medicine in the School of Medicine at the State University of New York at Stony Brook, was a virtual nonexerciser until he was forty-four years old and found himself breathing heavily after walking up a flight of stairs. He came to walking after embarking on a self-designed marathon-running program and participating in triathlons. While alternately running and walking through most of the final 26.2-mile running segment of the 1985 Cape Cod Endurance Triathlon, Jonas found that he hurt when he ran and felt much better when he walked quickly. He began to devise what he now calls PaceWalking.

"PaceWalking is essentially walking, but at a brisk and continuous pace to elevate the heart rate," says Dr. Jonas. In 1987 and 1988, Jonas PaceWalked the New York City Marathon, and in the process, passed hundreds of struggling runners.

Since the primary goal of walking is to improve health through aerobic exercise, Jonas believes that the key to PaceWalking is to elevate the heart rate for a minimum of twenty minutes three times a week. If you want to be scientific about your walking, you can take your pulse regularly every five or ten minutes as you walk, picking up the pace or slowing down depending on how you feel. In lieu of taking your pulse, you can use common sense while observing your exertion. If you're walking fast and generating a little body heat, then you most likely are within the lower limits of exercise intensity. If you're breathing hard and it's a struggle to continue, then you've pushed to your upper limits. When you're walking, try to pace your breaths: two steps, inhale, three steps, exhale, or any combination that works best for you.

Basic Equipment

While fitness walking—moving along at a speed of four miles per hour with one and a quarter times your body weight coming down at each footfall—doesn't demand special shoes, Dr. Rippe notes that any time there has been an attempt to stretch the limits of an activity, technology has risen to make it more pleasurable and safe.

"Is there anyone who doubts that the modern ski boot is better today than fifteen years ago? Or that the modern tennis racket is better than the wooden ones? The same goes for walking shoes," says Rippe. "In my way of thinking, the only piece of equipment that a serious walker must have is a pair of comfortable shoes made especially for walking."

Dr. Rippe advises that when you are looking for walking shoes, be sure that they have the following: a firm heel counter that will "cup" the heel and keep it from moving in the shoe; leather or leather-and-nylon-mesh uppers that will provide support and ventilation; light weight; a comfortable toe box (the front of the shoe) that will allow the toes to spread out comfortably as you walk; a thick, well-cushioned heel area to support the foot as it hits the ground; and a specific design that takes into account the walking stride.

Also pay attention to the socks you wear. Dr. Jonas recommends either 100 percent cotton or blends of cotton and a synthetic like orlon. "The job of socks is to cushion your feet and also to keep them dry," says Jonas. "There's nothing more uncomfortable during a walk than cold, wet feet."

Walking Technique

Walking for fitness doesn't require any special technique. "You just walk at a faster pace than normal without having to learn the exaggerated motion of race walking," says Rippe.

Anybody can get an aerobic workout from walking, that is, getting the heart rate to at least 60 percent of its maximum capacity and holding it there for twenty minutes. Says Rippe, "Our research points out that by increasing one's regular walking speed from three miles per hour to four miles per hour, the typical adult can easily get his heart rate into the target zone."

Four miles an hour won't cause many physically fit adults to break into a sweat, and walking at this pace is hardly a workout for someone with a moderate level of fitness. However, for someone who's been inactive for quite some time, four mph will provide a good workout. "In our studies of young marathoners," explains Rippe, "it was found that in order to get their heart rates up to the appropriate level, they had to walk a little faster than five miles per hour." When Rippe fitness-walks, he moves at speeds between five and a half mph and six mph, easily getting his pulse from a resting rate in the mid-40s up to his target range of 135 beats per minute.

Hand-held weights and weighted belts are regularly sold to walkers who are looking to get a better workout, but Dr. Rippe does not favor this practice. "The beauty of walking is in its simplicity," he says. "In our society, as soon as you get something simple, people want to make it more complicated. I have no problem with people wanting to incorporate weights into their walks after they've been walking for at least six months, but my own advice to these people would be to forget the weights and just walk faster or else include hills in their walking route."

Walking Tips

Walking can be more pleasurable with some careful preparation. According to Dr. Steven Jonas, anyone who has asthma and hasn't been exercising before should consult his or her physician and discuss plans to begin a walking program. After you get the green light to begin, your walking will be enhanced if you:

- Stretch before your walk, with emphasis on the muscle groups of your legs and back.
- Warm up and cool down properly. The best warm-up is to start out walking very slowly, gradually increasing your intensity. For your cool-down, gradually reduce your walking

intensity in the last five minutes until you reach your resting pulse rate.

- Maintain a regular, comfortable stride.
- Keep your back straight and your head level. Look ahead. Focus on a point off in the distance.
- Take deep, rhythmic breaths from your belly.
- Land on the outside corner of your heel, rolling forward on the outside edge of the foot, then pushing off with all your toes at the same time.
- Bend slightly at the hips; bending at the waist cramps the diaphragm and hinders breathing.
- Swing your arms back and forth with closed fingers for balance and rhythm. On the forward swing each hand should reach just above the waist. The back swing should stop when you feel your shoulder muscles start to stretch.

Suggested Training Program

As for all successful training programs, a plan should be laid out for your weekly walking program. This program should provide you with attainable goals and should allow your body to adapt comfortably to the exercise so you can make steady gains.

Walking for fitness usually means a pace of three to four miles an hour (one mile for every fifteen to twenty minutes). If this is too strenuous, or if you feel pain in your legs or feet or your breathing becomes labored, slow down to a more comfortable pace. "There is nothing wrong with walking slowly," says Dr. Rippe. "Everyone has to start somewhere."

On Walk One of your workout week, an easy walk for a beginner could be 20 minutes long, while a more fit walker could go out for approximately 30 minutes. On Walk Two, the novice can increase the pace slightly and stretch the duration to approximately 30 minutes; the fit walker could go for 45 minutes to an hour. On a weekend or other day when you have plenty of time, a long walk at a steady and rhythmic pace is appropriate, 60 minutes for the novice, 30 minutes longer for the fit walker.

Suggested Walking Schedule

Day	Walk Type	Beginner	Intermediate
Day 1	Easy walk	20 minutes	30 minutes
Day 2	Medium walk	30 minutes	45 minutes
Day 3	Rest	—	—
Day 4	Easy walk	30 minutes	45 minutes
Day 5	Medium walk	45 minutes	60 minutes
Day 6	Long walk	60 minutes	Up to 90 minutes
Day 7	Rest	—	—
TOTAL WALK TIME		140 minutes	210 minutes

THE ROCKPORT FITNESS WALKING TEST

The Rockport Fitness Walking Test is one of the most accurate tests of cardiovascular fitness and is an easy way for you to assess your current fitness level. Developed by Dr. James Rippe and his associates at the exercise physiology laboratory at the University of Massachusetts Medical School, the test has no significant limitations in terms of vigor, ease, or injury risk, and, best of all, you can get a clear idea of just how fit you are.

Instructions on how to take the test are reprinted on the pages that follow.

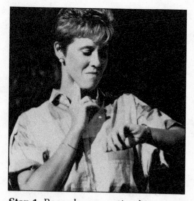

Step 1. *Record your resting heart rate.* If you do not know how to take your heart rate, use the following procedure. Walk in place for 30 seconds, then place your second and third fingers softly into the side of your neck at the level of the Adam's apple. Count your pulse for 15 seconds and multiply it by four to determine the rate per minute.

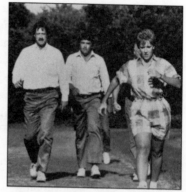

Step 2. *Find a measured track or measure out a mile of your own, and then walk a mile as fast as you can.* Before you begin, make sure to stretch properly, wear a good pair of walking shoes and loose-fitting clothing.

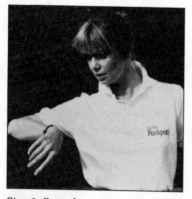

Step 3. *Record your time precisely at the end of the mile.* Since walking speeds vary greatly, you may want to try this more than once to make sure your first mile time is not inaccurate.

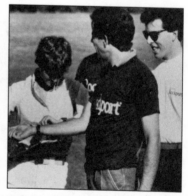

Step 4. *Record your heart rate immediately at the end of the mile.* With your recorded time, this will give you all the information you need to know to determine your level of fitness and an exercise program.

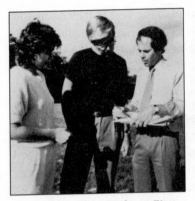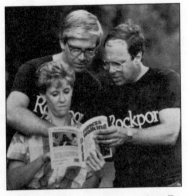

Step 5. *Turn to the Rockport Fitness Walking Test charts for your age and sex marked Relative Fitness Level and Exercise Program. Mark the point on the Relative Fitness Level chart defined by your walking time and heart rate to compare your results with individuals of your age and sex. Then look at the same point on the Exercise Program chart to determine your program.*

Step 6. *Turn to your appropriate Exercise Program chart and begin your twenty-week walking program. Repeat the Rockport Fitness Walking Test at the end of the twenty weeks.*

(Courtesy of the Rockport Walking Institute, copyright © 1986 by The Rockport Company)

Find Your Fitness Level

1. Turn to the "Relative Fitness Level" chart on pages 197–199 appropriate for your age and sex. This chart shows the relative fitness level of other people of your age and sex according to established fitness norms from the American Heart Association.

2. Mark the point on the chart defined by your walking time and heart rate at the end of the walk. This allows you to compare your performance to those of others in your age and sex category.

3. Next, look at the appropriate letter-coded "Exercise Program" chart for your age and sex. Again, mark your coordinates on this chart. Note the letter area that you fall in.

4. Turn to the program on pages 200–202 that corresponds to the letter area you were in on the Exercise Program chart. Start the program outlined for your level and follow it for twenty weeks.

5. Repeat the Rockport Fitness Walking Test at the end of your twenty weeks. This will determine your fitness level and whether or not you should advance to a new workout.

RELATIVE FITNESS LEVEL CHARTS

These charts are designed to show you how fit you are compared with other individuals of your age and sex. For example, if your coordinates place you in the "Above Average" section of the chart, you're in better shape than the average person in your category.

The charts are based on weights of 170 pounds for men and 125 pounds for women. If you weigh substantially more, your relative cardiovascular fitness level will be slightly overestimated. If you weigh substantially less, your relative cardiovascular fitness level will be slightly underestimated.

EXERCISE PROGRAM CHARTS

By using the same coordinates as you did on the Relative Fitness Level charts, you can use these charts to determine which exercise program you should follow.

Again, go along the horizontal axis ("Time") until you reach the point that represents how long it took you to walk the mile. Then follow the vertical axis to the coordinate representing your pulse rate. Note the letter of the section where these two coordinates meet and turn to the exercise program corresponding to that letter.

Relative Fitness Level and Exercise Program Charts

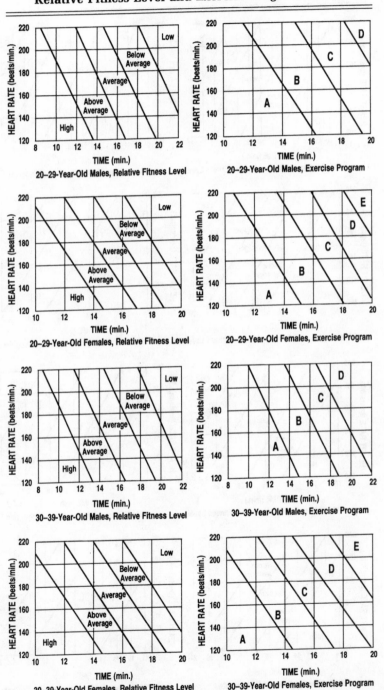

20–29-Year-Old Males, Relative Fitness Level

20–29-Year-Old Males, Exercise Program

20–29-Year-Old Females, Relative Fitness Level

20–29-Year-Old Females, Exercise Program

30–39-Year-Old Males, Relative Fitness Level

30–39-Year-Old Males, Exercise Program

30–39-Year-Old Females, Relative Fitness Level

30–39-Year-Old Females, Exercise Program

Relative Fitness Level and Exercise Program Charts

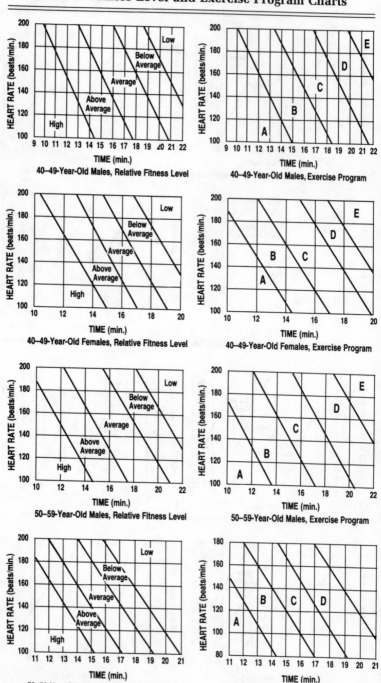

40–49-Year-Old Males, Relative Fitness Level

40–49-Year-Old Males, Exercise Program

40–49-Year-Old Females, Relative Fitness Level

40–49-Year-Old Females, Exercise Program

50–59-Year-Old Males, Relative Fitness Level

50–59-Year-Old Males, Exercise Program

50–59-Year-Old Females, Relative Fitness Level

50–59-Year-Old Females, Exercise Program

Relative Fitness Level and Exercise Program Charts

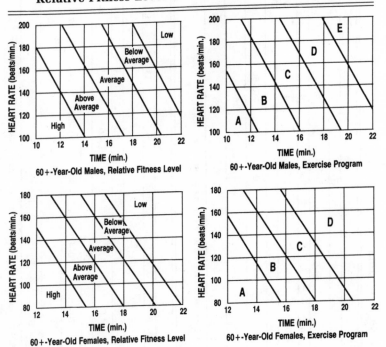

(Courtesy of the Rockport Walking Institute)

The Exercise Programs

The Rockport Walking Programs are designed to help maintain or improve your level of fitness, depending on your current level. For optimal results, follow the programs closely.

On each program there are columns labeled "Pace" and "Heart Rate." The pace listed is only an approximation. Walking speed should be determined by the pace that keeps your heart rate at the appropriate percentage of maximum listed.

At the end of the twenty-week period, retake the Rockport Fitness Walking Test to determine your new fitness level and exercise program.

Exercise Programs

A PROGRAM

WEEK	1	2	3	4	5	6	7–20
WARM-UP (mins. before walk stretches)	5–7	5–7	5–7	5–7	5–7	5–7	5–7
MILEAGE	3.0	3.25	3.5	3.5	3.75	4.0	4.0
PACE (mph)	4.0	4.0	4.0	4.5	4.5	4.5	4.5
INCLINE/WEIGHT							+
HEART RATE (% of max.)	70	70	70	70–80	70–80	70–80	70–80
COOL-DOWN (mins. after walk stretches)	5–7	5–7	5–7	5–7	5–7	5–7	5–7
FREQUENCY (times per week)	5	5	5	5	5	5	3

At the end of the twenty-week fitness walking protocol turn to the A/B Maintenance Program for a lifetime of fitness walking.

B PROGRAM

WEEK	1	2	3–4	5	6	7	8	9–10	11–14	15–20
WARM-UP (mins. before walk stretches)	5–7	5–7	5–7	5–7	5–7	5–7	5–7	5–7	5–7	5–7
MILEAGE	2.5	2.75	3.0	3.25	3.25	3.5	3.75	4.0	4.0	4.0
PACE (mph)	3.5	3.5	3.5	3.5	4.0	4.0	4.0	4.0	4.5	4.5
INCLINE/WEIGHT										+
HEART RATE (% of max.)	70	70	70	70	70–80	70–80	70–80	70–80	70–80	70–80
COOL-DOWN (mins. after walk stretches)	5–7	5–7	5–7	5–7	5–7	5–7	5–7	5–7	5–7	5–7
FREQUENCY (times per week)	5	5	5	5	5	5	5	5	5	3

At the end of the twenty-week fitness walking protocol follow the A/B Maintenance Program for a lifetime of fitness walking.

C PROGRAM

WEEK	1	2	3–4	5	6–8	9–10	11–12	13–14	15	16–17	18–20
WARM-UP (mins. before walk stretches)	5–7	5–7	5–7	5–7	5–7	5–7	5–7	5–7	5–7	5–7	5–7
MILEAGE	2.0	2.25	2.5	2.75	2.75	3.0	3.0	3.25	3.5	3.5	4.0
PACE (mph)	3.0	3.0	3.0	3.0	3.5	3.5	4.0	4.0	4.0	4.5	4.5
HEART RATE (% of max.)	70	70	70	70	70	70	70–80	70–80	70–80	70–80	70–80
COOL-DOWN (mins. after walk stretches)	5–7	5–7	5–7	5–7	5–7	5–7	5–7	5–7	5–7	5–7	5–7
FREQUENCY (times per week)	5	5	5	5	5	5	5	5	5	5	5

At the end of the twenty-week fitness walking protocol, you may either retest yourself and move to a new fitness walking category or follow the C Maintenance Program for a lifetime of fitness walking.

D PROGRAM

WEEK	1–2	3–4	5–6	7	8–9	10–12	13	14	15–16	17–18	19–20
WARM-UP (mins. before walk stretches)	5–7	5–7	5–7	5–7	5–7	5–7	5–7	5–7	5–7	5–7	5–7
MILEAGE	1.5	1.75	2.0	2.0	2.25	2.5	2.75	2.75	3.0	3.25	3.5
PACE (mph)	3.0	3.0	3.0	3.5	3.5	3.5	3.5	4.0	4.0	4.0	4.0
HEART RATE (% of max.)	60–70	60–70	60–70	70	70	70	70	70–80	70–80	70–80	70–80
COOL-DOWN (mins. after walk stretches)	5–7	5–7	5–7	5–7	5–7	5–7	5–7	5–7	5–7	5–7	5–7
FREQUENCY (times per week)	5	5	5	5	5	5	5	5	5	5	5

At the end of the twenty-week fitness walking protocol, retest yourself to establish your new program.

E PROGRAM

WEEK	1–2	3–4	5	6	7–8	9	10	11	12–13	14	15–16	17–18	19–20
WARM-UP (mins. before walk stretches)	5–7	5–7	5–7	5–7	5–7	5–7	5–7	5–7	5–7	5–7	5–7	5–7	5–7
MILEAGE	1.0	1.25	1.5	1.5	1.75	2.0	2.0	2.0	2.25	2.5	2.5	2.75	3.0
PACE (mph)	3.0	3.0	3.0	3.5	3.5	3.5	3.75	3.75	3.75	3.75	4.0	4.0	4.0
HEART RATE (% of max.)	60	60	60	60–70	60–70	60–70	60–70	70	70	70	70	70–80	70–80
COOL-DOWN (mins. after walk stretches)	5–7	5–7	5–7	5–7	5–7	5–7	5–7	5–7	5–7	5–7	5–7	5–7	5–7
FREQUENCY (times per week)	5	5	5	5	5	5	5	5	5	5	5	5	5

At the end of the twenty-week fitness walking protocol, retest yourself to establish your new program.

A/B MAINTENANCE PROGRAM

WARM-UP: 5–7 minutes before walk stretches

AEROBIC WORKOUT: mileage: 4.0; pace: 4.5 mph weight/incline: add weights to upper body or add hill walking as needed to keep heart rate in target zone (70–80% of predicted maximum)

HEART RATE: 70–80% of maximum

COOL-DOWN: 5–7 minutes after walk stretches

FREQUENCY: 3–5 times per week

WEEKLY MILEAGE: 12–20 miles

C MAINTENANCE PROGRAM

WARM-UP: 5–7 minutes before walk stretches

AEROBIC WORKOUT: mileage: 4.0; pace: 4.5 mph

HEART RATE: 70–80% of maximum

COOL-DOWN: 5–7 minutes after walk stretches

FREQUENCY: 3–5 times per week

WEEKLY MILEAGE: 12–20 miles

(Courtesy of the Rockport Walking Institute)

RUNNING

Running is one of the quickest routes to cardiovascular fitness. World-class runners generally have the most developed hearts and lungs of any group of athletes (including cross-country skiers, cyclists, swimmers, and oarsmen) and often have a lower percentage of body fat as well.

Perhaps the greatest advantage to building your fitness program around running is its convenience. With a good pair of shoes, you can run day or night, throughout all four seasons. The world is your track: the beach, an empty golf course, a city street, a country road. When the weather is bad, you can run up stairs, run in place, or run on a treadmill.

Running exerts tremendous force on the body. When you run, each foot-strike exerts the force of two to four times your body weight on your skeleton. Starting at your feet, this jarring sensation moves up through the shin, the knee, hips, back, and eventually ends at your head. Therefore, in order to minimize running injuries and increase your running enjoyment, it's essential to have a good pair of running shoes. The days of the twenty-five-dollar running shoes are over, so expect to pay anywhere from fifty to one hundred dollars. Choose shoes that are comfortable. The shoe sole shouldn't be too stiff and your toes shouldn't be cramped or pinched. Be sure the heel counter (the back of the shoe that helps control the rear foot during running) is stiff and holds your heel firmly in place.

Each footfall should start with the heel or midsole hitting first. Roll forward and then push off with the ball of the foot. If you land on the ball of your foot first, you risk straining the bones in the front of the foot as well as the calf muscles.

Running Technique

The best way to run is the way that feels most natural for you. While there are no set rules regarding proper running form, there are certain generalities that, if followed, will help you to run faster, longer, and more efficiently.

Posture plays an important part in distance running. Once your foot is on the ground, imagine that there is a straight line running from your foot through your hips up your back to your shoulders and head. Your center of gravity should be right along this line, with just a hint of a forward lean. If you happen to lean too far forward past this line when you run, or too far to the rear, you will become biomechanically inefficient, wasting both motion and energy. Analysis of the world's top runners reveals that the almost straight-up running style is the most efficient way to run.

When you run, try to run relaxed, though you may find this difficult when you're working through a five-miler and feel exhausted. However, by relaxing your arms and unclenching your hands, concentrating on a smooth and fluid stride, you'll get the most out of your workout.

Your arms should be in sync with your body as you run. Ideally, your arms should be carried high and close to your chest, the elbows bent at a ninety-degree angle. Don't flap your arms or cross them in front of you. As you run, your arms should move back and forth, each arm moving in sync with the opposite leg. Your hands should almost touch your hips as you go. Avoid clenching your fists into tight balls, which will result in a stiff running style. Instead, keep your fingers extended and slightly bent, with the index fingers gently touching the thumbs.

Running Distances

One of the most important things to remember in starting a running program is to start slowly. You may plan to run a marathon eventually, but you'll need more than a year to prepare properly. If you want to run a 10K race, it could take almost a half year of hard training. Have patience.

If you're new to running, don't go hard your first time out. Pick a shorter distance than what you actually feel like running and alternate several minutes of jogging with brisk walking until you cover it. For the first several weeks of your program, be sure to alternate running with a slower-paced jog or brisk walk. Over time, increase the length of your running segment until you can comfortably run the entire distance without stopping.

One of the major causes of injury to runners is that they take too big an increase in their training distances without letting their bodies first adapt to the stresses that distance running brings on. A beginner might go from a one-mile to a two-mile workout and experience little difficulty. But go from, say, five miles up to ten miles, and you may be in for trouble. Running experts agree that jumps of 10 percent in mileage each week are acceptable and relatively safe. Push your mileage past this safety guideline and you're asking for trouble.

The best guide to how much mileage you should run is your body. Aches and pains should alert you that you're running too hard or too far. If you begin wheezing or have trouble breathing, don't try to push through it. Slow down and assess the situation. Do you need more medication? Should you end the workout for now? Trying to push through your asthma sounds heroic, but you may pay the price of impaired health.

BICYCLING

Bicycling is booming: ninety million people are expected to be riding each year, for recreation, in competition, and for fitness. Bicycle vacations and tours are becoming popular, and more people are finding that they can combine their exercise with practicality by riding their bike to work instead of taking the car. Yes, all of this is possible even if you have asthma.

"I find cycling to be challenging, both mentally and physically," says Marion Clignet. The Olney, Maryland, cyclist reached national-class level after training with her bike for only two years.

Clignet has asthma, as well as epilepsy, but she successfully manages both with a carefully monitored medication program. "I love to compete," says Clignet, "and nothing is going to hold me back." Clignet now trains year-round and sometimes rides over seventy-five miles a day. Her dedication paid off in 1988 when she was selected to race nationally with the highly regarded Ten Speed Drive racing team.

Cycling a multigear bike several times a week is great for cardio-respiratory fitness. In one study comparing running to cycling during a twenty-week span, cycling was found to be just as effective a conditioner as running. And cycling offers the benefits of running without the high levels of fatigue and muscle soreness.

Climatic conditions may pose problems for cyclists with asthma. If your asthma is triggered by cold air, wearing a mask around the nose and mouth may help. Airborne pollen can be particularly problematic because of the different environments a cyclist can pass through on a long ride. "Being totally aware of your triggers and where you have to ride is all that you can really do," says Clignet. "If the pollen or air pollution gets to be too bad, you have to retreat indoors and train on a stationary bike."

Top athletes from other sports are drawn to cycling because of its gentle movement. Bill Walton, the former Boston Celtic center, was an avid cyclist throughout his pro basketball career, and he owns many bicycles custom-built to accommodate his 6 foot 11 frame. Marty Liquori, at one time the fastest 5,000-meter runner in the world, took up cycling and now competes in races throughout Florida. "The beauty of cycling," says Liquori, who now runs three days a week and cycles on the other days, "is that you can push yourself as hard as you can on the bike and the next day you can go out and hammer away again. On the other hand, after a running race your body shows signs of wear and tear and you have to take some time off to recuperate."

If there is a downside to cycling it lies in its potential for danger. Even the most careful cyclist can be surprised by a dog, confronted with a gaping hole in the street, or brushed by a poorly driven car. Accidents do happen, often resulting in "road rash" and broken bones. Be sure to wear an approved bike helmet, even if you're just going to the store to pick up some milk.

Cycling has legions of adherents. With the ability to charge up hills and then coast back down, to see more changing scenery in a day than a runner ever will in a week, and to vary workouts simply by changing gears, once you become a cyclist, you're usually hooked for life.

COMMON BEGINNER MISTAKES

Mistakes on your bike can lead to injury. The most common include:

- Trying to ignore asthma and push through a workout while wheezing and hacking. As you should during other aerobic activities when you feel asthma coming on, slow down if you have to (stopping completely can actually aggravate asthma in some cases) and assess your asthma. If you need your inhaler, use it before continuing with your workout. There are no trophies or ribbons given for seeing how long you can go without medication.
- Turning the pedals slowly while in a high gear. This puts too much strain on the delicate knee joints. Select a gear in which you can comfortably pedal between 80 and 110 revolutions per minute.
- Going too far, too fast, too soon. This will leave you sore all over. Take it easy until you're able to build up necessary muscle strength. As your fitness progresses, increase your pedaling cadence and distance.
- Riding in a straight-up position. This is an inefficient way to ride, especially in a headwind; 75 percent of your energy will be spent just trying to overcome air resistance. For top riding efficiency and comfort, bend from the waist into a tuck position.

EQUIPMENT

Buying a Bike

You can use any type of bike for exercise. However, a 12-speed racing or touring frame bike or an 18-speed mountain bike is better suited to both hills and flat terrain than the typical 3-speed bike. Prices for bikes vary, anywhere from $300 for a good entry-level bike to $2,000 for a top-of-the-line racing model.

"Go to a good pro bike shop for the best advice, the best bikes, good service, and, most important, a good fit," says Marion Clignet. "Like a pair of comfortable shoes, a bike frame has to fit your body frame properly. If something is off in sizing you're eventually going to develop problems with your knees or back."

Clothing

The proper clothing will make your workouts more enjoyable. Snug-fitting Lycra shorts help prevent your bottom and thighs from chafing and offer the best protection from saddle sores. A soft chamois lining on the inside of the crotch absorbs perspiration, reduces friction, and helps cushion you on your ride. Their prices range from $20 to $75.

Jerseys should be form-fitting to allow you maximum freedom of movement. Try on the jersey in the store, making sure that it's long enough in the back to keep you covered when you're bent over the handlebars. Prices are usually $15 to $50.

A good pair of cycling shoes with cleats or ones fitted with a special plastic insert for new pedal binding systems will enhance pedaling efficiency by 30 percent to 40 percent (because they allow you to push down *and* pull up on the pedals), minimize fatigue, and help prevent foot and leg cramps. Expect to pay between $25 and $100.

Wear a Helmet

Each year there are more than one thousand cyclists killed in the United States, 75 percent of whom die from injuries to the head. "I wear my helmet at all times," says Marion Clignet, who trains more than 400 miles a week and races on most weekends of the year. "A fifty-dollar helmet investment is the best one you'll ever make for yourself." There are now dozens of helmet brands on the market. Check that the one you buy has been tested and approved by either the American National Standards Institute (ANSI) or the Snell Memorial Foundation.

SUGGESTED TRAINING PROGRAM

If you're just a beginner, it's best to start out cycling slowly, according to John Howard, a two-time Olympic cyclist from Encinitas, California. Howard recommends that for the first month you cycle 20 minutes at a time, three times a week (every other day is best), on a flat course that is as free of cars as possible. In a 20-minute ride you should be able to cover approximately three miles. "Keep your gears in the midrange in order to keep yourself from straining your knees," says Howard.

By your second month, increase your cycling frequency and duration. Push your cycling time up to a half hour and add another day to your schedule. A long ride on the weekend is recommended. Hill riding can also be introduced. By your third month, your legs and lungs should be ready for a faster pace.

Suggested Cycling Schedule

Month	Short-Ride Mileage	Long-Ride Mileage
1	3–6	5–12
2	4–8	10–20
3	7–10	20–40
4	9–14	Up to 50

A good way to train is to ride with others. Joining a cycling club and participating in their group rides and workouts will help you assess your strengths and weaknesses while providing you with friendly companionship.

16

AEROBIC DANCE

In recent years, many people have been lured back to exercise by aerobic dance. It offers low-impact dance steps (the dancer keeps at least one foot on the floor at all times to reduce stress to the joints) plus the fun of exercising in a group. The beauty of aerobic dance is that for many people it's more of a social occasion than exercise. Many people who take up aerobic dance don't even realize they're exercising, but after several weeks they make tremendous fitness gains.

While class settings encourage people to exercise harder and are generally more fun, aerobic dance can also be done in the privacy of your own home by following videotaped workouts on your VCR.

Aerobics for Asthmatics is a low-impact aerobics tape that I developed in conjunction with two asthma specialists (available from Aerobics for Asthmatics, Inc., 10301 Georgia Avenue, Suite 306, Silver Spring, MD 20902, 301-681-6055). This forty-five-minute exercise video is designed specifically to help people with asthma improve their cardiovascular system, strengthen the muscles that control breathing, and improve their exercise tolerance. Many people who have used this tape over the last several years

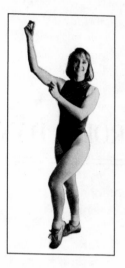

have reported good fitness gains. Others have used the tape for a few months to learn about their bodies and about exercising with asthma, and then have gone on to use the skills taught in the tape in other sports such as tennis and soccer.

HOW TO GET STARTED

Aerobic dancing is certainly enjoyable, but it is important that you understand that it is first and foremost an aerobic exercise. Just like swimming, brisk walking, and bicycling, aerobic dance must be performed regularly several times a week at a level that will elevate your pulse for at least fifteen to twenty minutes. Merely moving around to music will not make you fit.

A good aerobic dance program involves the muscles of the torso, arms, and legs, boosting the heart rate to a level of exertion at which you'll start to develop cardiorespiratory fitness and holding it there for at least twenty minutes. Benefits of aerobic dance include reduction of body fat, improved flexibility, and increased muscle endurance. You can specifically focus your movements to develop the muscle groups of the chest, back, and abdomen, which is critical in improving your respiratory fitness.

For someone with asthma, low-impact aerobics is an effective way to get fit. It can even be combined with other aerobic exercises such as swimming or brisk walking, adding to your overall fitness and keeping your exercise week varied, challenging, and pleasurable.

Aerobic dance can bring on its share of injuries if you're not careful. Stress injuries and muscle pulls are common for beginners because of the variety of movements they have to perform. In general, these injuries are minor and are cured easily with rest.

Reading a book about aerobic dance is not a good way to get started exercising because it's difficult to pick up good dance routines by looking at the pictures. Therefore, it's a good idea to start an aerobics dance program with a good aerobics video or in an organized class under the supervision of a qualified instructor. The better instructors are certified by one of two dance organizations, either Aerobics Fitness Association of America (AFAA) or International Dance Exercise Association (IDEA). These trained professionals know how to provide the basics to help you safely build a sufficient level of stamina. After several weeks of practice, you can begin to perform your own workout at home.

EQUIPMENT

Proper shoes are the most important piece of equipment needed for aerobic dance. A well-designed aerobic shoe is cushioned in the forefoot to protect the balls of your feet when you land. Expect to pay $30 to $75 for a good pair.

A proper dance surface is also important because it will reduce the impact when your feet come down. A wooden floor suspended several inches over the actual floor is ideal. Concrete or a rug over concrete is the worst surface to dance on and is not recommended.

BEGINNING A WORKOUT

Aerobic dance can be strenuous, so each class should begin with a gradual buildup of movement and intensity to allow the joints and muscles to become accustomed to the demands. If at any time during a workout you get fatigued or feel asthma starting to come on, slow down. Some people find that moving slowly in place until the asthma passes allows them to rejoin the class very quickly without having to go through an entire warm-up routine once again. Don't feel bad about using your inhaler if you have to. A few puffs and you can often be back with the class in no time.

It's important that you pay close attention to your body alignment as you go through your routines. If you try to perform a movement with bad posture it can lead to an injury.

Music, of course, is the key to aerobic dance workouts. It should have a steady rhythm that will inspire you to move. Make sure that there are no sudden jumps in tempo. Going abruptly from a slow pace to a frenetic beat will exhaust you quickly, and may cause muscle strain.

If you'll be doing your exercising at home, choose your music carefully. Your warm-up should have slow music, while the aerobic phase should be relatively fast-paced and continuous for at least fifteen to twenty minutes. As you cool down, the music should be slow-paced to gradually reduce your activity level.

APPENDIX A

ASTHMA CAMPS

There are many benefits to sending your child to an asthma summer camp. The emphasis is always on fun, and the children take part in the typical camp fare of sports, arts and crafts, nature study, and theater just like any other children. However, children with asthma are taught at camp that they can do what they think they can't. It's this important lesson that most of them carry home with them.

Although homesickness is often a problem for children at first, being away from parents (some of whom are understandably over-protective) gives them a sense of independence and makes them more aware that they are responsible for their medication. Parents benefit, too, by learning to let go of their child. They also get a little more time to spend with other children in the family and with their spouses.

When deciding on a camp, make sure that the camp has a *resident physician* on staff and is close to a hospital. If there is not a camp listed in your area, call your local branch of the American Lung Association for a referral. The following is a national list of summer camps for children with asthma (from the American Academy of Allergy and Immunology).

NAME	LOCATION	DIRECTOR

Arizona

Camp Not-A-Wheeze
Ages: 8–13

Friendly Pines

Arizona Asthma
  Foundation
3310 West Bell Road
Phoenix, AZ 85023

Arkansas

Camp Aldersgate
Ages: 7–16

Little Rock

Camp Aldersgate, Inc.
2000 Aldersgate Road
Little Rock, AR 72205
Director: Diane
  Barnes

California

Southern California
  Asthmatic Medical
  Program
Ages: 9–14

Running Spring

Geoff Stephens
Mary Ellen Friedman,
  M.D.

Scamp Camp
Ages: 9–14

William Wallace,
  M.D.
765 Academy Drive
Solana Beach, CA
  92075

AAFA Summer
  Asthma Camp
Ages: 8–12

Boys Club Camp 369,
  Running Spring

Asthma and Allergy
  Foundation of
  America: LA
  Chapter
5410 Wilshire
  Boulevard, #1015
Los Angeles, CA
  90036

ALA of Los Angeles
Ages: 8–14

Running Spring

American Lung
  Association of Los
  Angeles County
Mr. Robert E. Field
5858 Wilshire
  Boulevard
Los Angeles, CA
  90036–0926

NAME	LOCATION	DIRECTOR

Camp Superstuff
Ages: 6–10
	Day camp at
	  California State
	  University, Fresno
		American Lung
		  Association
		PO Box 11187
		Fresno, CA 93772

Sierra Asthma Camp
Ages: 11–14
	Camp Sequoia,
	  Kings Canyon Park
		American Lung
		  Association of
		  Central California
		PO Box 11187
		Fresno, CA 93772
		Director: Wendell
		  Boone

Colorado

Champ Camp
Ages: 7–14
	Woodland Park,
	  Estes Park
		Tony Marostica
		1119 West 6th Street,
		  #100
		Pueblo, CO 81003

Champ Camp
Ages: 7–14
	Woodland Park	Colorado Allergy
		  Society
		William S. Silvers,
		  M.D.
		7180 East Orchard
		  Road
		Englewood, CO 80111

Champ Camp
Ages: 7–14
	YMCA Camp at
	  Rocky Mountain
	  National Park
		Colorado Allergy
		  Society
		William S. Silvers,
		  M.D.
		7180 East Orchard
		  Road
		Englewood, CO 80111

NAME	LOCATION	DIRECTOR

Florida

Sunshine Station Camp
Ages: 7–11
		Barry D. Dusch
		Director of
		  Community and
		  Child Education
		American Lung
		  Association
		Fort Lauderdale, FL
		  33316

Sunshine Station Camp
Ages: 7–11
		American Lung
		  Association of
		  Florida
		PO Box 8127
		Jacksonville, FL
		  32239

Georgia

Camp Breathe Easy
Ages: 8–15
	Cleveland	American Lung
		  Association of
		  Atlanta
		723 Piedmont Avenue
		  NE
		Atlanta, GA 30365–
		  0701

Hawaii

Hawaii Asthma Camp
Ages: 7–12
		Franklin Y.
		  Yamamoto, M.D.
		99128 Aiea Heights
		  Drive, #107
		Aiea, HI 96701

Idaho

Camp Lutherhaver
Ages: 6–12
	Coeur d'Alene, ID	American Lung
		  Association of
		  Washington
		North 1322 Ash,
		  Spokane, WA 99201
		Director: Sara
		  Swanson

NAME	LOCATION	DIRECTOR

Illinois

| Camp AAFA
Ages: 8–13 | Camp Ravenwood,
Lake Villa | Asthma and Allergy
Foundation of
America
Greater Chicago
Chapter
111 North Wabash,
#909
Chicago, IL 60602
Director: Lou Katz,
R.N. |

Iowa

| Camp AAFA
Ages: 7–16 | Des Moines YMCA
Camp | American Lung
Association of Iowa
1321 Walnut
Des Moines, IA 50309
Director: Laurie Alber |
| Camp Superkids
Ages: 7–16 | Des Moines YMCA
Camp | Dr. Edward Nassif
McFarland Clinic
Ames, IA 50010 |

Massachusetts

| Camp Chestnut
Ages: 8–14 | The Warren Center,
Ashland | American Lung
Association of
Essex County
239 Newburyport
Turnpike
Topsfield, MA 10983 |

Michigan

| Camp Sun Deer
Ages: 9–12 | Battle Creek Outdoor
Education Center,
Dowling | American Lung
Association of
Southeastern
Michigan
28 West Adams
Detroit, MI 48226
Cynthia Ramsey, R.N. |

NAME	LOCATION	DIRECTOR

Camp Michi-Mac
Camp Nissokone
Ages: 10–15
	Oscoda	Allen Sosin, M.D.
		23023 Orchard Lake
		   Road
		Farmington, MI 48024
		
		David Seaman, M.D.
		8578 North Canton
		   Center
		Canton, MI 48187

Camp Michi-Mac
Camp Ohiyesa
Ages: 7–10
	Holly	Allen Sosin, M.D.
		23023 Orchard Lake
		   Road
		Farmington, MI 48024
		
		David Seaman, M.D.
		8578 North Canton
		   Center
		Canton, MI 48187

Minnesota

Camp SUPERKIDS
Ages: 7–14
	YMCA Camp
	   Ihdulhapi,
	   Loretto
		American Lung
		   Association of
		   Hennepin County
		1829 Portland
		   Avenue
		Minneapolis, MN
		   55404

Montana

Camp Huff and Puff
Ages: 7–10
	West: Lion's
	   Sunshine Camp,
	   Elliston
	
	East: Bear Mountain
	   Ranch, Dean
		American Lung
		   Association
		825 Helena Avenue
		Helena, MT 59601
		1-800-252-6368

Nebraska

Camp Superkids Ages: 7–14		Linda B. Ford, M.D. 401 East Gold Coast Road, #107 Papillion, NE 68128

NAME	LOCATION	DIRECTOR

New Hampshire

| Camp Super Kids
Ages: 7–14 | YMCA Camp
Coniston,
Grantham | Lily Yee
New Hampshire Lung
Association
PO Box 1040
Manchester, NH
03105 |

New Jersey

| Ocean Cruises | Mexico, Bermuda,
Canada | Gerry Comeau
The Respiratory
Health Association
55 Paramus Road
Paramus, NJ 07652
201-843-4111 |

New Mexico

| Stephen Lopez
Memorial Camp for
Asthmatic Children
Ages: 9–16 | Camp Summer Life,
near Taos | Billie Dytzel
American Lung
Association of New
Mexico
216 Truman NE
Albuquerque, NM
87108 |
| Camp Superkids
Camp Superteens
Ages: 9–16 | Camp Summer Life,
near Taos | American Lung
Association of New
Mexico
216 Truman NE
Albuquerque, NM
87108 |

New York

| Camp SUPERKIDS
Ages: 7–13 | Old Forge | American Lung
Association of Mid-
New York
2323 South Street
Utica, NY 13501
Director: Mary
Fogarty, M.D. |

NAME	LOCATION	DIRECTOR
North Dakota		
Dakota Superkids Ages: 8–15	Triangle YMCA Camp, Sakakawea	American Lung Association of North Dakota 212 North 2nd Street PO Box 5004 Bismarck, ND 58502 Director: Marcie Andre
Ohio		
Camp SUPERKIDS Ages: 7–14	Camp Allyn, Batavia	American Lung Association of Southwestern Ohio 2330 Victory Parkway Cincinnati, OH 45206
Oklahoma		
Camp Green Country Ages: 7–15	Camp Waluhili, Wagoner	American Lung Association of Green County 5553 South Peoria Tulsa, OK 74105
Texas		
Camp Sunshine Ages: 8–12	Dallas	Ms. Carolyn Crawford American Lung Association PO Box 190625 Dallas, TX 75219–9990 William R. Lumry, M.D. 5499 Glen Lakes Drive, #100 Dallas, TX 75231

NAME	LOCATION	DIRECTOR

Virginia

Camp Holiday Trails
Ages: 7–14

Charlottesville

Dr. Elsa Paulsen
PO Box 5806
Charlottesville, VA
22905

Wisconsin

Camp Wikidas
Ages: 8–14

Wisconsin Dells

American Lung
Association of
Wisconsin and
Wisconsin Allergy
Society
1 South Park Street,
#600
Madison, WI 53715–
1393

APPENDIX B

RESOURCES

Treatment Centers for Severe Asthma

The following centers offer treatment for severe asthma.

Asthmatic Children's Foundation of New York
PO Box 568
Spring Valley Road
Ossining, NY 10562
914-762-2110

The foundation operates a residential treatment center for children ages five to fifteen with severe asthma. Questions about asthma are answered and referrals are also offered.

National Foundation for Asthma/Tucson Medical Center
5301 East Grant Road
Tucson, AZ 85712
602-323-6046

Operates an outpatient clinic, supports research, and publishes informative asthma booklets for the public.

National Jewish Center for Immunology and Respiratory Medicine
1400 Jackson Street
Denver, CO 80206
303-388-4461

National Jewish is the nation's top research, treatment, and education facility for asthma and other respiratory conditions. The facility accepts chronic asthma patients from around the country on referral from physicians. The center makes physician referrals, publishes many asthma booklets, and staffs the toll-free LUNG LINE (1-800-222-LUNG). In Colorado, call 303-388-4461.

Organizations

The following organizations offer printed materials, answer questions about asthma, sponsor community workshops, and can often refer you to local asthma support groups, physicians specializing in asthma, and summer asthma camps.

American Academy of Allergy and Immunology
611 East Wells Street
Milwaukee, WI 53202
414-272-6071

Asthma and Allergy Foundation of America
1717 Massachusetts Avenue, NW, Suite 305
Washington, DC 20036
202-265-0265

American Lung Association
1740 Broadway
New York, NY 10019
212-315-8700

Lung Line
1-800-222-LUNG; in Colorado, 303-398-1477; within the Denver
metropolitan area, 303-355-LUNG

Call 8:30 A.M. to 5:00 P.M. MST to ask any asthma-related question or to
request asthma booklets.

Mothers of Asthmatics, Inc.
10875 Main Street, Suite 210
Fairfax, VA 22030
703-385-4403

Books

Asthma: Stop Suffering, Start
    Living
M. Eric Gershwin, M.D., and E. L.
    Klingelhofer, M.D.
Addison-Wesley ($10.95,
    paperback)

Asthma: The Complete Guide for
    Patients and Their Families
Allan M. Weinstein, M.D.
McGraw-Hill ($17.95, hardcover);
    Fawcett ($4.95, paperback)

Breathing Easy: A Handbook for
    Asthmatics
Genell Subak-Sharpe
Doubleday ($17.95, hardcover)

Children with Asthma: A Manual
    for Parents
Thomas F. Plaut, M.D.
Pedipress, Inc.
125 Red Gate Lane
Amherst, MA 01002
($9.95, paperback; order by mail,
    prepaid)

The Essential Asthma Book: A
    Manual for Asthmatics of All
    Ages
Francois Haas, Ph.D., and Sheila
    Sperber Haas
Charles Scribner's Sons ($16.95,
    hardcover)

Parent's Guide to Asthma
Nancy Sander
Doubleday ($17.95, hardcover)

Newsletters

Asthma & Allergy Advocate
American Academy of Allergy and
    Immunology
611 East Wells Street
Milwaukee, WI 53202
414-272-6071
(four issues, $5 per issue)

MA Report
Nancy Sander
Mothers of Asthmatics, Inc.
10875 Main Street, Suite 210
Fairfax, VA 22030
703-385-4403
(12 issues, write for rates
and a free sample)

Asthma Today
Leo Leonidas, M.D.
412 State Street
Bangor, ME 04401
207-947-6739
(12 issues, $20)

APPENDIX C

MEDICATION CONTAINING SULFITES

Over the years serious adverse reactions have been associated with the use of sulfiting agents (sodium sulfite, sodium and potassium metabisulfite, and sulfur dioxide) in various products. Sulfites are present in a substantial number of asthma-related drug products. If you are sulfite-sensitive, be sure to check this list before using a medication to determine whether the product contains sulfites.

I. Bronchodilator Inhalant Solutions

Arm-A-Med (Isoetharine hydrochloride)

Arm-A-Med (Metaproterenol Hydrochloride)

Asthmanefrin Solution (Racemic epinephrine)

Bronkosol (Isoetharine HCl) 1% Solution

Bronkosol 0.25% Unijet

Bronkosol Unit Dose

Isoetharine HCl 0.125%, 0.062%, 0.167%, 0.200%, and 0.25%

Isoproterenol HCl 0.62%, 0.031%

Isuprel Hydrochloride Solution (Isoproterenol HCl) 1:100, 1:200 Solution

Metaprel (Metaproterenol sulfate) Solution 5%

Micronefrin (Racemic epinephrine)

Vapo-Iso Solution (Isoproterenol HCl)

Vaponefrin Solution (Racepinephrine)

II. Syrups and Tablets

Aldomet Oral Suspension

Aminophyllin Tablets

Anacin-3 Tablets

227

Aspirin-Free Arthritis Pain Formula Tablets

Aspirin-Free Dristan AF Tablets

Children's Chewable Anacin-3 Tablets

Clisten D Tablets

Codeine Tablets

Colrex Compound Elixir

Decadron LA Suspension

Dextroamphetamine Sulfate 5 and 10 mg Tablets

Elixophyllin-K1 Elixir

Fer-In-Sol Drops and Syrup

Isuprel Compound Elixir

Isuprel HCl Glossets (10, 15 mg)

Maximum Strength Anacin-3 Tablets

Metaprel Syrup

Methyldopa Tablets 250 mg and 500 mg

Moban Concentrate

Parafon Forte Tablets

Soma Compound With Codeine

Tacaryl Hydrochloride Syrup (Methdilazine HCl)

Talacen Tablets

Trendar Tablets

Tylenol Acetaminophen With Codeine Capsules

Tylenol Acetaminophen With Codeine Tablets

Tylox Oxycodone and Acetaminophen Capsules

X-Trozine 35 mg Tabs Yellow, Green

III. Injectables

Adrenalin 1:1000 (Epinephrine)

Aldomet Ester HCl Injection (Methyldopate HCl MSD)

Antilirium Injection

Aramine (Metaraminol Bitartrate)

Atropine With Demerol Injection Carpuject (50, 75 mg)

Bronkephrine (Ethylnorepinephrine HCl injection)

Carbocaine 2% With Neo-Cobefrin Inj. Carpules

Celestone Phosphate (Brand of Betamethasone Sodium)

Chlorpromazine HCl Injection, U.S.P. 25 mg/ml Tubex

Citanest Forte 4% Solution With Epinephrine 1:200,000

Codeine Phosphate Injection, U.S.P. 30 mg/ml and 60 mg/ml tubex

Compazine (Prochlorperazine) Ampuls

Decadron LA Suspension (Dexamethasone Acetate)

Decadron Phosphate Injection (Dexamethasone Sodium Phosphate)

Decadron Phosphate With Xylocaine (Dexamethasone Sodium Phosphate & Lidocaine HCl)

Dexamethasone Sodium Phosphate Injection tubex

Dopamine Hydrochloride Injection

Dopastat (Dopamine HCl)

Duranest 0.5 Solution with Epinephrine 1:200,000

Epinephrine Injection (USP)

EpiPen, EpiPen Jr.

Hexadrol Injection

Hydeltrasol Injection

Hydrocortone Injection

I-131 Iodohippurate Injection

I-131 Serum Albumin Human Injection

Intropin (Dopamine HCl)

Isoproterenol HCl Injection, U.S.P.

Isuprel HCl Sterile Injection 1:5000 (Isoproterenol HCl) Ampul

Largon (Propiomazine HCl) 20 mg/ml tubex

Levophed Bitartrate (Norepinephrine Bitartrate) 0.1% Inj ampul

Levoprome (Methotrimeprazine)

Lidocaine HCl 1 & 2% With Epinephrine

Marcaine (0.25, 0.50, 0.75%) with Epi Inj. Ampul

Marcaine (0.25, 0.50, 0.75%) with Epi Inj Vial

Marcaine HCl (0.5%) With Epinephrine (Bupivacaine HCl & Epinephrine) Inj. Carpul

Mepergan (Meperidine & Promethazine HCl) Injection Tubex

Meperidine HCl Injection 50 mg/ml-30 ml vial and 100 mg/ml-20 ml vial

Metaraminol Bitartrate Injection

Morphine Sulfate Injection Carpuject (2, 4, 8, 10, 15 mg)

Neo-Synephrine 1% Injection Ampul

Nesacaine 1 & 2% Solution (Chloroprocaine HCl)

Nesacain-CE 2 & 3% Solution (Chloroprocaine HCl)

Norflex Injectable

Novocain (Brand of Procaine HCl) 1%, 2%, and 10% Injection Ampul

Nubain (Nalbuphine HCl)

Phenergan (Promethazine HCl) 25 mg/ml, 50 mg/ml

Pontocaine 1% Solution Injection Ampul

Procaine HCl

Promethazine HCl

Pronestyl (Procainamide HCl) 100 mg/ml, 500 mg/ml

RNL Injectable Carpules

RNN Injectable Carpules

Ru-A-Dron (Prednisolone Sodium Phosphate)

Ru-Phen (Promethazine HCl)

Sensorcaine Solutions with Epinephrine 1:200,000 for Infiltration & Nerve Block

Serpasil (Reserpine USP)

Sparine Injection 25 mg/ml, 50 mg/ml, tubex

Stelazine Multi-Dose Vials

Synkayvite Injectable (Menadiol Sodium Diphosphate)

Talwin Injection Vial 30 mg and Carpuject (30, 45, 60 mg)

Tensilon Injectable Solution

Thorazine (Chlorpromazine HCl) Ampuls and Multi-dose Vials

Tofranil (Imipramine HCl USP) Ampuls, 25 mg per 2 ml

Torecan (Brand of Thiethylperazine maleate USP)

10% Travasol (Amino Acid) Injection Without Electrolytes

Trilafon (Brand of Perphenazine USP)

Tubocurarine Chloride Injection USP

Vasoxyl Injection

Xylocaine Solutions (Lidocaine HCl) with Epinephrine 1:200,000

Yutopar (Ritodrine HCl)

IV. Antibiotics

Amikin (Amikacin Sulfate) Injection

Apogen for Injection

Bactrim IV Infusion (Trimethoprim and Sulfamethoxazole)

Bristagen (Gentamicin Sulfate) Injection

Gantrisin (Sulfisoxazole) Injection

Garamycin Injectable (Gentamicin Sulfate)

Gentamicin Sulfate Injection

Kantrex Injection (Kanamycin Sulfate)

Klebcil for Injection

Minocin Syrup (Minocycline Hydrochloride)

Mysteclin-F Syrup (Tetracycline and Amphotericin)

Nebcin (Tobramycin Sulfate) Injection

Septra IV Infusion

Sumycin Syrup (Tetracycline)

Topicycline Solution

Vibramycin Syrup (Doxycycline Calcium)

V. Miscellaneous

A. *Nose Drops or Sprays*

Alconefrin 12, 25, 50 drops

Alconefrin 25 spray

Allerest Nasal Spray

Sinarest Nasal Spray

B. *Eye Drops*

Decadron in Ocumeter

Decadron Phosphate—0.1% Sterile Ophthalmic Solution (Dexamethasone Sodium Phosphate)

Epifrin 0.25%, 0.50%, 2.0% Sterile Ophthalmic Solution

Eserine 0.5% (Steri unit, i.e. 2 ml unit)

Isopto Eserine 0.25% and .5%

Murocoll—2 Ophthalmic Solution

Mydfrin 2.5% Ophthalmic Solution

Neodecadron Sterile Ophthalmic Solution (Neomycin Sulfate—Dexamethasone Sodium Phosphate)

Pred-Forte Ophthalmic Suspension

Pred-Mild Ophthalmic Suspension

Prefrin-A Sterile Ophthalmic Solution

Prefrin-Z Sterile Ophthalmic Solution

Propine Ophthalmic Suspension

Sulfrin Ophthalmic Suspension

C. *Ear Drops*

Cortisporin Otic Solution (Polymyxin B-Neomycin-Hydrocortisone)

Drotic Otic Solution

Otocort Ear Drops

Tympagesic Otic Solution

D. *Suppositories*

Summer's Eve Vaginal Suppositories

E. *Topical Creams, Ointments, Lotions, and Gels*

Caldecort Cream

Carmol H C Cream

Dibucaine Ointment

Eldopaque Cream

Eldopaque Forte Cream

Eldoquin Cream

Eldoquin Forte Cream

Eldoquin Lotion

Lasan Cream

Neodecadron Topical Cream

Pabanol Lotion

Pontocaine 1% Cream

Postacne Lotion

Rezamid Lotion

Solaquin Cream

Solaquin Forte Cream

Solaquin Forte Gel

Sulfacet-R Lotion

Sulfamylon Cream

Vitadye Lotion

INDEX